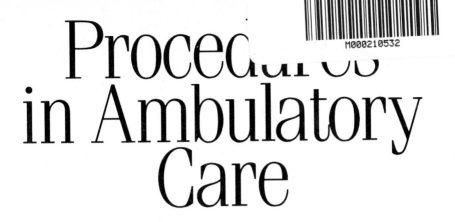

Procedures in Ambulatory Care

Robert D. Gillette, M.D.

St. Elizabeth Family Health Center
Youngstown, Ohio
Formerly, Department of Family Medicine
University of Cincinnati
College of Medicine

McGraw-Hill Book Company

New York   St. Louis   San Francisco   Auckland   Bogotá   Caracas   Colorado Springs
Hamburg   Lisbon   London   Madrid   Mexico   Milan   Montreal   New Delhi
Oklahoma City   Panama   Paris   San Juan   São Paulo   Singapore   Sydney
Tokyo   Toronto

PROCEDURES IN AMBULATORY CARE

Copyright © 1987 by McGraw-Hill, Inc. All rights reserved. Printed in the United States of America. Except as permitted under the United States Copyright Act of 1976, no part of this publication may be reproduced or distributed in any form or by any means, or stored in a data base or retrieval system, without the prior written permission of the publisher.

1 2 3 4 5 6 7 8 9 0 HAL HAL 8 9 4 3 2 1 0 8 7

ISBN 0-07-023265-2

This book was set in Times Roman by the McGraw-Hill Book Company Publishing Center in cooperation with Monotype Composition Company. The editors were William Day and Stuart D. Boynton; the production supervisor was Elaine Gardenier; the designer was Jules Perlmutter, Off-Broadway Graphics.
Arcata Graphics/Halliday was the printer and binder.

Library of Congress Cataloging-in-Publication Data

Gillette, Robert D.
  Procedures in ambulatory care.

  Includes bibliographies and index.
  1. Family medicine—Handbooks, manuals, etc.
2. Primary medical care—Handbooks, manuals, etc.
I. Title. [DNLM: 1. Ambulatory Care—methods.
2. Community Health Services—organization & administration. 3. Primary Health Care—methods. W 84.6 G479p]
RC55.G55 1987   616   87-2655
ISBN 0-07-023265-2

Contents

List of Consultants

BRADLEY BUSACCO, M.D.
Assistant Professor of Clinical
   Obstetrics/Gynecology
Department of Obstetrics/
   Gynecology
University of Cincinnati

JOHN W. DAVREN, M.D.
Assistant Clinical Professor
Department of Family Medicine
University of Cincinnati

ANDREW T. FILAK, JR., M.D.
Assistant Professor
Department of Family Medicine
University of Cincinnati

RICHARD S. MORAITES, M.D.
Assistant Clinical Professor
Department of Dermatology
University of Cincinnati

LUIS E. QUIROGA, M.D.
Clinical Instructor
Department of Family Medicine
University of Cincinnati

MICHAEL D. SCHAEN, M.D.
Associate Professor of Clinical
   Family Medicine
Department of Family Medicine
University of Cincinnati

DAVID N. TUCKER, M.D.
Ophthalmologist
Cincinnati, Ohio

ELMER F. WAHL, M.D.
Assistant Clinical Professor
Department of Family Medicine
University of Cincinnati

Foreword

Ambulatory care, the major emphasis of family practice and a significant component of other primary care disciplines, is now accepted as a most important aspect of our changing modern health care system. The increasing scientific literature on the subject is a healthy sign which bodes well for the future. With advice from family physician colleagues and other specialists with whom he works, Dr. Gillette has selected and described procedures which he considers essential and basic to good modern primary care practice. His work describes practical and convenient ways of improving and adding to the range of services available to our office patients, thus adding to the completeness of ambulatory/primary care practice. The book is readable and will be welcomed by residents as they prepare for their future careers. It will also be valued by more seasoned practitioners as a convenient reference, reducing the need to search through larger texts. The office nurse will also find much of interest and direct applicability to her activities.

The author brings together a vast amount of helpful clinical information derived from many years of experience as a practicing family physician and teacher. His familiarity with the territory can be easily recognized in these pages. His approach is that of a caring physician who keeps his patients' interests paramount. Apart from cost-effectiveness and convenience to the patient, well-done procedures confer a sense of fulfillment and satisfaction on the practitioner. The role of the primary physician in our health care system is strengthened, and depersonalization and fragmentation of service, two of the major negative features of health care, are minimized.

We are grateful to the author for the effort and care he has given in the preparation of this very useful book. To cover procedures in primary care practice is a daunting challenge. Choices had to be made and I believe that Dr. Gillette and his colleagues have used excellent judgment in selecting the areas that really matter. They deal in a succinct, practical way with most of what is likely to be required of the primary physician. Their contribution is timely and welcome.

Robert Smith, M.D.,
Professor and Director
Department of Family Medicine
University of Cincinnati

Preface

Since the work of family physicians and other providers of primary care is defined largely by the problems presented by their patients, they should be educated and equipped to perform a number of frequently-indicated patient care procedures. Family medicine's primary *raison d'être* is its orientation to the needs patients are most likely to have, its goal that of providing "uncommonly good care for common problems." Minor lacerations, anal symptoms, ocular foreign bodies, and other problems calling for hands-on treatment appear frequently, and we should be ready to care for them. This book has been designed to meet the need for a single resource containing information about procedures that can and should be performed in medical offices and other unspecialized ambulatory care facilities. It is intended to be a useful tool in daily practice, not a decoration or a doorstop. It should acquire thumbprints and perhaps coffee stains as it is used by resident physicians and others to learn procedures and by experienced practitioners to review their fine points. It is directed primarily at physicians, but nursing and other staff personnel involved with procedures may find it of value.

Subject matter has been selected on the basis of personal experience, advice from numerous capable consultants, and review of the medical literature. To be included, a procedure must be done commonly, be relatively simple to perform and suitable for ambulatory practice, carry reasonably low risk of complications, and have a good prognosis when properly executed. A physician considers many factors in deciding whether to treat a problem or refer it. Can it be managed with the personnel and facilities available? Does the practitioner do the procedure often enough to be good at it? How much discomfort will there be for the patient? How great is the risk of a bad outcome? How much inconvenience and delay will the patient face if the problem is referred to a subspecialist? Family doctors should not hesitate to perform low-risk procedures which appear frequently in their practices, whether or not they seem to belong to the "turf" of one subspecialty or another. If a practitioner can perform a procedure as well as anyone else, he or she ought to do it if only to save the patient the inconvenience and cost of having to go elsewhere. If a subspecialist can get a significantly better result with lower risk of adverse effects, the patient's interest calls for a referral. Wanting to do a procedure in the primary care office should never be an excuse for taking unnecessary chances with a patient's well-being.

The choice and description of specific methods are based on review of standard textbooks, recent medical literature, and the experiences of the author and consultants. They reflect a synthesis of input from both community and academic practice. This process has required some decisions which are not supported by, and occasionally conflict with, the recent medical literature. Some of what has been published in this area is biased by specialty interests. Techniques have been described which are too complex and too costly in relation to the problems for which they are advocated (ingrown toenails, for example). In some subject areas the author and consultants have chosen to depart from that which appears in print and to advocate time-tested simple forms of treatment in preference to alternatives which are more impressive but give no better final results.

A quarter century of medical practice has taught the author to respect and work with the body's natural forces and to avoid interventions that interfere with the healing process. As a result there is a bias in this book for thinking in physiological rather than mechanical terms and for avoiding further insult to injured tissues. These approaches have proved effective in providing high quality care to patients at reasonably low cost, and readers will find them useful in their own practices. Complexity and high cost do not necessarily indicate care of superior quality.

My sincere thanks to all my consultants, both those listed and other colleagues in the University of Cincinnati College of Medicine who gave informal advice on the structure and wording of the text, for their valuable contributions. The artwork of Stan Coffman and Lisa McElravy of the University of Cincinnati's Medical Center Information and Communications Department is also appreciated. Although the advent of word processing has greatly diminished the tedium of typing and retyping drafts, Kathy Emerson and Kathy Slone contributed greatly to the logistical aspects of the project, and I am grateful to them. Ruth Kraus, R.N., Director of Nurses of UC's Family Practice Center, deserves thanks for patiently answering dozens of questions about equipment, supplies, and procedures. Thanks, too, to the Family Health Foundation of America and to the University of Cincinnati's Medical Center Library for providing the extensive bibliographic services needed for a book with subject matter as diverse as this one.

Robert D. Gillette, M.D.

chapter 1

Approach to the Patient

In a busy medical practice there is a frequent temptation to focus on procedures and neglect the people on whom they are done. This may have adverse consequences for both patient and practitioner. A patient who is anxious because of misinformation or a misunderstanding may experience unnecessary pain. One who has not been instructed in aftercare, or who was instructed in a way that didn't "sink in," may have a poor end result. A physician who conveys the image of being uncaring, inept, or distracted may have difficulty attracting and keeping patients.

PUTTING YOURSELF IN THE PATIENT'S PLACE

It's often useful to make a conscious effort to view medical care from the patient's perspective. Imagine, for example, that you have recently moved to a new community and need a physician's services because of a painful perianal mass. A neighbor recommends a family practice nearby, and you call for an appointment. You are pleased that the person with whom you talk on the telephone asks only enough questions to determine the urgency of your problem and offers the earliest available appointment. When you arrive, you are greeted by name, but no mention of the nature of your illness is made within earshot of others. The facility is neat and clean, and staff members convey an aura of caring and competence. If you will have to wait for more than a few minutes because your physician is busy with another patient, you are given a reasonably honest estimate of the length of the delay and offered a cup of coffee.

You are ushered into a tidy, well-equipped examining room, and your initial interview with the doctor occurs while you are still fully dressed. Enough questions are asked to elicit the nature of your illness and any possible complicating problems, although a detailed history may be deferred until the cause of your pain has been addressed. Examination reveals a thrombosed external hemorrhoid. The doctor explains the nature of the lesion, reassures you about its benign prognosis, and outlines the options for treatment. Your questions are answered in lay terms, and the doctor listens to be sure you have assimilated the information.

You feel that the severity of your pain justifies excision of the mass and so inform the physician. The risks of local anesthesia are explained, but without frightening you unnecessarily. Under the guidance of an aide you assume the necessary position. The practitioner warns you to expect the momentary pain of the hypodermic needle and then proceeds with the operation. All needed equipment and supplies are at hand, ready for use. The aide monitors your pulse and blood pressure and carries on a light conversation with you. In less than an hour after you walked in the door, you walk out again, feeling better both because your pain has been relieved promptly and because you were comfortable with the physical surroundings and the people who cared for you. You were called by name, listened to, and treated as an adult worthy of respect.

Achievement of this ideal is not always easy. Patients can be abrasive, sometimes intentionally and sometimes inadvertently. Physicians and their staffs work under significant professional and time pressures, and sometimes they must cope with personal pressures as well. The managerial support needed for a practice to function smoothly is not always forthcoming. However, taking extra effort to meet the standards described above pays dividends. Patients tell their friends and neighbors when they have been treated well, and hostile, abrasive people become more mellow when they feel they can get attention and care without acting unpleasant.

WORKING WITH SMALL CHILDREN

The approach to children begins in the waiting room, one section of which should have small tables and chairs, some durable and easily washed toys, perhaps a blackboard and chalk, an assortment of children's books and magazines, and something for them to watch. Some favor television sets, but others find them noisy and distracting for adults nearby. An aquarium is a pleasant addition which children of all ages will enjoy, provided someone on the staff takes care of it regularly.

In an examining room a child will tend to cling to the parent until he or she feels reasonably safe. This should be encouraged. Indeed, most of a physical examination can be conducted with the patient on the parent's lap. Watch your "body language" around children: Smile. Let the patient become accustomed to your presence before doing anything painful or threatening. If possible, sit or kneel so your face is near the child's level. Avoid hurried speech or movements. Call the child by name. Explain what you're going to do in simple terms. Choose nonthreatening words; if you say, "This won't hurt much," the child is likely to hear only the word "hurt." Be careful that the tone and inflection of your voice are calm and reassuring.

Children welcome the opportunity to demonstrate their abilities, and it's sometimes appropriate to exploit this tendency. "I'll bet you can climb up on that examining table all by yourself" is sometimes a useful gambit. Those who work with children soon learn many other little games that make things pleasanter for everyone concerned.

When a painful procedure is necessary, start by telling the child and parent what is going to happen, giving reassurance that you will be very careful and cause as little discomfort as possible. Set up all necessary staff and equipment before disturbing the child, and then get the task over with as quickly as possible. Once it is completed, let the parent comfort the patient, compliment the child on having cooperated so well, and perhaps give him or her a small reward as a distraction.

We often think of parents as "second patients," and with good reason. If they are anxious or distracted, their children may sense this and become frightened. Parents may have feelings of inadequacy or guilt when their children are sick and fear being criticized by medical personnel. Complimenting them on the care they have given their youngsters or acknowledging how difficult it can be to work with sick children may relieve these feelings, reduce anxiety, and open the way for more pleasant and productive patient care encounters.

chapter 2

Surgical Principles and Technique

No surgery is "minor" in the eyes of the surgeon, the patient, or the law. Carelessness in even the most minor operation carries significant risks. Both patients and the courts expect that ambulatory surgery will be done in properly equipped facilities by well trained, alert, and highly motivated people. Many operative procedures can be carried out safely in medical offices and other ambulatory facilities if due caution is observed. The situation may be compared to a mine field for which an accurate map is at hand: One who moves with care and follows the map precisely will do well.

Each practice must decide for itself what procedures to perform, considering such factors as the education and skills of the physicians, the patient population being served, time and financial constraints, and the availability of subspecialist services nearby. A practitioner in an isolated rural area who is interested in doing office surgery and has good manual skills will naturally do more than one less dextrous who functions in an urban multispecialty group.

EQUIPMENT AND SUPPLIES

Surgical equipment and supplies are available in many styles and forms, and there is room for individual preference. Some doctors use mostly disposables, while others prefer mostly durable purchases. Sterile paper draping sheets are readily available. They have the advantage of not requiring staff time for preparation and washing, but they are less flexible than cloth and tend to slide out of position easily. Sterile disposable scalpels are available for those who prefer them to disposable blades attached to reusable handles. Disposable suture removal sets are handy to use although the instruments are often crude.

Surgical instruments vary widely in price and quality. A busy practice may wish to invest in the best instruments available unless there is a high risk of theft or accidental disappearance. Some little used instruments may have to be purchased simply because it is impossible to know when they may be needed without advance notice (forceps for pharyngeal foreign bodies, for example). Some physicians prefer curved hemostats and scissors, while others are content with the slightly less expensive straight ones. Specific suggestions on scissors, hemostats, needle holders, tissue forceps, and other instruments are listed in chapter 19, "Equipment and Supplies."

Lidocaine (Xylocaine, other brands) is deservedly the most popular agent for local infiltration anesthesia. The 0.5% solution is strong enough for infiltration anesthesia and offers a wide safety margin. It may be stocked with and without epinephrine. The 1% solution is preferable for digital blocks; it should of course not contain epinephrine when used for this purpose. Bupivacaine (Marcaine, Sensorcaine) 0.25% solution can be stocked for procedures requiring anesthesia lasting longer than an hour. Ordinary plastic hypodermic syringes, readily available in different sizes, are satisfactory for most local infiltration anesthesia. Needles of about 20 gauge may be used to withdraw the agent from its vial. For infiltration 25-gauge needles are commonly used, but in the hands of a skilled operator, 27- or even 30-gauge needles are practical and will cause less discomfort for the patient.

Monofilament sutures of either nylon or polypropylene should be stocked in 4/0 and 5/0 sizes. Some operators can use 6/0 material comfortably, but many find it difficult to handle and easy to break. It may be helpful to stock both black (for easy visibility on light-skinned patients) and white (for dark-skinned patients) suture material. An absorbable suture material, 4/0 polyglycolate or perhaps plain gut, should also be on hand. These materials are supplied sterile in 18-inch lengths swaged to 3/8 circle-cutting needles.

Either disposable scalpels or scalpel blades will be required, #15 blades being satisfactory for most office surgery. Some operators may prefer #10 or possibly #11 blades for special purposes. The #12 blade, although not widely used, is an excellent choice for opening abscesses in most parts of the body (figure 2-1).

Dressing materials are available in a wide variety, and here again there is some room for individual preferences. Many of these products are best known by brand names, some of which will be listed for identification in the following paragraphs. No endorsement of the brands listed or criticism of those omitted is intended.

Skin closure strips such as Steri-strips can be used to close small wounds or to reinforce wounds when sutures have been removed early. The wider strips can also serve as primary dressings for small wounds.

Antistick products serve the useful role of preventing dressings from sticking to the skin. A small amount of serum will exude from even the most carefully sutured incision, "gluing" a gauze dressing to the skin as it dries. A material such as Telfa or one of the petrolatum-impregnated

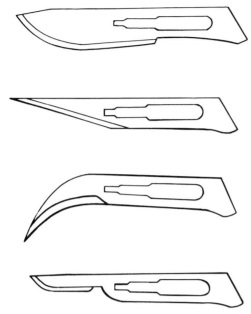

FIGURE 2-1
Surgical blades: #10, #11, #12, and #15.

fine-mesh gauze products such as Adaptic will prevent this problem, making it easier and less painful to remove the dressing at a subsequent visit.

Gauze sponges are used for many purposes, including skin cleansing, wiping away blood, and adding bulk to the dressing. The 3-inch-square size seems best suited to office practice, although larger and smaller sizes are available for those who prefer them.

Roller gauze may be used to hold dressings in place on the extremities. The one-inch size works well on fingers and toes. The two-inch and larger sizes may be preferred elsewhere. Proprietary tubular-gauze products make a neater-appearing dressing, although they must be stocked in a variety of sizes.

Aluminum splints come in various sizes and configurations. It is often desirable to incorporate them into dressings for immobilization and protection, especially with finger and hand lesions.

Adhesive tapes should be available in 0.5-, 1-, and 2-inch widths. Various materials are available to choose from. The traditional zinc oxide cloth type, despite its lower cost, is less preferable than the new products, except perhaps for taping joints.

Elastic bandages are used where compression of the injured area may be beneficial. They tend to slide out of position easily; this is less likely to happen with self-adherent products such as Coban. This product can also be cut into short lengths to make dressings for fingers or hands. With all elastic bandages one must be careful not to apply too much pressure; this is especially important with Coban, which has little tendency to sag in use.

WOUND HEALING

Understanding the factors which influence healing is essential to planning appropriate wound care (figure 2-2). A surgeon does not heal a laceration but simply creates an environment conducive to repair by closing it and protecting it from further insult until healing occurs. For practical purposes optimum healing can only occur if the following needs are met:

1. **Approximation of Tissues.** When the skin edges have been properly approximated, healing occurs rapidly and with minimum scar formation. When a gap occurs, the epithelium cannot bridge the defect until it has a fibrous tissue matrix on which to migrate; healing will therefore occur only after fibroblasts have laid down a bed of granulation tissue. The end result is delayed healing, excessive scar formation, and risk of infection and other forms of morbidity. The presence of dead space in the subcutaneous area is deleterious in two ways: First, serum will accumulate and infection may follow. Second, lack of support for the skin will lead to a cosmetically unsatisfactory depression in the surface contour.

2. **Healthy Wound Edges.** Optimum healing requires that the cells at the wound edge be vigorous and healthy. If irritating cleaning

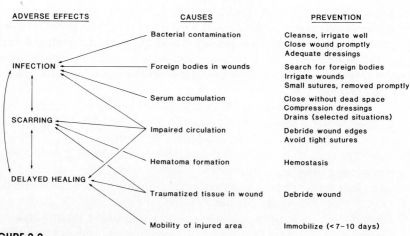

FIGURE 2-2
Causes of wound-healing problems.

solutions or antibacterial preparations come in contact with these cells, they may be damaged; therefore, strong solutions should not be permitted to get into the wound. Sterile isotonic saline is the irrigating solution of choice for most office surgery.

Excising traumatized wound edges is often desirable to promote prompt healing and minimal scar formation and to minimize the risk of infection. Debridement of devitalized subcutaneous tissues is useful for the same reasons.

Be gentle to the tissues. Do not crush them with rough use of tissue forceps; skin hooks are less traumatic. Keep the wound moist with normal saline if it is going to be open for more than a few minutes.

3. **Optimal Circulation to the Wound.** Nutrients must be readily available and antimicrobial factors must have ready access to the site if prompt healing is to occur. These requirements may not be met if the sutures are excessively tight ("approximate but do not strangulate") or if local circulation is otherwise impeded. For example, a bedridden patient with a lesion on a dependent part of the body may need to be turned frequently to avoid circulatory embarrassment from constant pressure on the site. Patients with large burns or other major injuries may need nutritional supplementation. Lesions on highly vascular areas such as the face typically heal more quickly and with less risk of complications than those on the extremities. Other important factors such as the age of the patient, general debility, and the presence of arterial insufficiency may be beyond the physician's control, but their presence may signal the need for extra caution in care of the patient.

4. **Freedom from Contamination.** The presence of foreign material or devitalized tissue in the wound may serve as a nidus for infection, and the presence of infection will retard or stop the healing process. These facts further underscore the importance of irrigating and debriding wounds (other than minor incised wounds) before closure. Suture materials are themselves foreign bodies, so absorbable materials should be employed beneath the skin and excessive amounts of suture material should be avoided.

Sterile technique is important to minimize the number of pathogenic organisms in the wound. It is practically impossible to accomplish perfect sterility in the ambulatory setting, but the fewer bacteria there are in the lesion, the less the risk that they will establish a foothold.

Antibiotics are not needed in minor wounds with good prognosis, but their use should be considered in major injuries with a high risk for infection. If possible, the first dose should be administered intravenously before other treatment is started. Prophylactic antibiotics should be discontinued two or at most three days after initial treatment. Further antimicrobial treatment is needed only if evidence of infection appears. Dressings play an important role in preventing wound contamination and infection. Their use will be discussed in a subsequent section in this chapter.

5. **Immobilization.** Injuries heal best and are least susceptible to infection when they are immobilized. Depending on the nature of the problem, this can be accomplished with bulky dressings, splints, bed rest, or other specific techniques. However, immobilization also carries risks, including loss of muscle tone, joint stiffness, and at the extreme thromboembolism. The extent and duration of immobilization is determined by balancing these considerations as well as such additional factors as convenience and cost to the patient.

STERILE TECHNIQUE

Most ambulatory settings do not permit the level of sterile technique employed in a hospital surgical suite. Caps, masks, and surgical gowns are generally not worn, and space limitations may require the office surgery room to be utilized also for casting, endoscopy, and other procedures. This is acceptable if high-risk operations are avoided and if everyone involved has a "sterile conscience" and acts accordingly.

The basic principles of sterile technique are taught to all medical and nursing students, but enough carelessness is seen in day-to-day practice that we have chosen to review them here. An object which has been sterilized (made free of dirt and microorganisms) must not be allowed to touch anything which is not equally sterile. If accidental contamination occurs, the contaminated object is immediately removed from the operative site, or if this is impossible, it is covered with a sterile drape. A common example is accidentally letting the tail of a piece of suture drag over an undraped surface. If only the end of the suture is contaminated, the operator can snip off the unsterile end and let it fall to the floor. If more of the suture is compromised, it should be discarded completely.

Donning sterile gloves requires adherence to the same principle. Start by opening the package carefully, being sure that the flap you have touched does not spring back and contaminate the gloves. Touch only the *Inside* of the first glove you put on (figure 2-3), and then using the gloved hand, touch only the *Outside* of the second glove (figure 2-4). Get in the habit of holding your gloved hands in plain sight in front of you, and don't hesitate to change gloves if one accidentally touches an unsterile object.

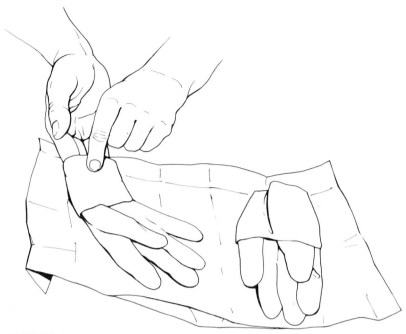

FIGURE 2-3
Donning the first glove.

Most sterile supplies come in containers which are intended to be opened without touching the contents. The intent is that the suture pack, dressing, or other sterile object will drop freely onto the draped Mayo stand, ready for use. In actual practice many of the packages are poorly designed, so that contamination of their contents occurs easily. Also, many dressings and other light objects tend to stick to the packaging and must be pulled loose with sterile forceps. There are two ways to deal with these problems. One is to use great care in removing sterile objects from their packages. The other is to purchase unsterile supplies, package them properly, and autoclave them on site.

The presence of airborne contamination cannot be prevented completely in most medical offices, but a number of commonsense precautions can and should be followed. Good housekeeping techniques will minimize airborne dirt. Avoid fans or heating systems that can stir up dust. Abscesses and other gross infections should not be treated in a room where sterile procedures will be done. If a series of unanticipated wound infections should occur, the staff should be cultured to identify carriers of staphylococci or other pathogens.

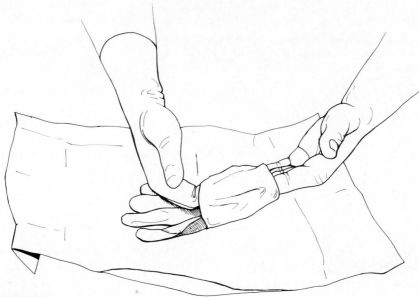

FIGURE 2-4
Donning the second glove.

MANUAL SURGICAL SKILLS

One needs a combination of knowledge and manual skills to perform surgical procedures quickly, neatly, and with minimal damage to tissue. Dexterity is gained by practicing on simulation devices (Ethicon Company, other sources), pigs' feet, broiler chickens, and even grapefruit. Continue the learning process by monitoring the results of your work in your patients: Did a wound become infected? Did it heal promptly and with the smallest possible scar? Was normal function restored completely?

Scalpels should be grasped as you would a pen for the best possible control for small surgical procedures. The heel of the hand and the little finger should lie on the patient (if practical) to stabilize the hand. Hold the blade perpendicular to the skin (as viewed from above) so that the edges of the incision will come together smoothly. For the finest scar, incline the scalpel no more than 10 degrees so that the wound edges will be slightly everted when apposed (figure 2-5). Make firm, confident strokes with the scalpel to avoid jagged, irregular incisions. Stretch the skin and hold it taut with the opposite hand when making an incision.

Hemostats are held with the thumb in one loop of the instrument and the middle or ring finger in the other. The tip of the index finger rests on

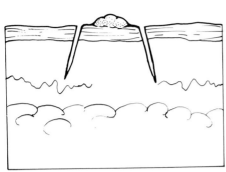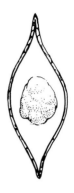

FIGURE 2-5
Incline elective incisions slightly for best cosmetic results.

or near the hinge to provide maximum control of the tip of the instrument (figure 2-6). Apply the hemostat as precisely as possible to the bleeding point, crushing as little tissue as possible. Avoid at all costs the urge to grasp blindly when the field fills with blood; the risk of damaging vital structures is high. It is much safer to control bleeding with direct pressure until the problem can be assessed and its solution planned.

Scissors are held the same way as hemostats. They should seldom be used to cut skin but are often appropriate for dissection of softer

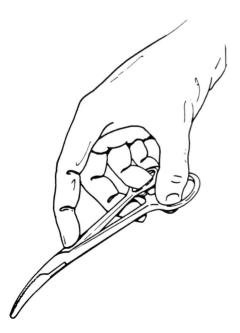

FIGURE 2-6
Method of holding hemostat.

subcutaneous tissues. Scissors and hemostats are easily damaged by being put to uses for which they are not designed.

Needle holders come in an endless variety of sizes, tips, and style of locks. There are even needle holders with built-in scissors; they are suitable only for minor procedures which do not involve buried sutures or fine detail. There is a tendency to use needles that are too short and to compensate by grasping them at the weak swaged end. This leads to bending and breaking. Needles should be grasped about a third of their length from the swaged end.

Tissue forceps may be used (gently) where cosmetic appearance is not crucial. The Adson type or others with multiple fine teeth are preferred. For the best in atraumatic wound care, manipulate the skin only with *skin hooks*.

Gauze sponges should be used only with a gentle dabbing motion. Wiping living tissue with gauze sponges is traumatic and tends to dislodge fresh clots.

KNOT TYING

Variations of the square knot are used for almost all ambulatory surgery. For buried sutures, where it is important to minimize the volume of foreign material, use the simple two-level square knot (figure 2-7); place the knot at the bottom of the suture loop as described in the section on excision of skin and subcutaneous masses. (See Chapter 3.) The monofilament suture materials employed in skin closure are relatively slippery; use an extra turn in the first knot to prevent slipping (surgeon's knot), and use a total of four knots (figure 2-8).

Where the skin must be closed under some tension, it is sometimes useful to make a knot that can be gradually tightened. To do this, tie a square knot loosely and then pull one end of the suture out straight to invert ("dump") the knot (figure 2-9). When tightened, this knot is strong enough only for temporary use in approximating the wound edges. Once the appropriate amount of tension has been achieved, tie another square knot on top of it.

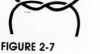

FIGURE 2-7
Square knot.

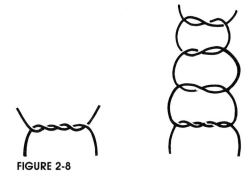

FIGURE 2-8
Surgeon's knot.

The instrument method is preferred for most knot tying in the primary care setting. It can be done quickly and wastes little suture material. The method is shown in figure 2-10. Skill with one-handed or two-handed knot tying should also be developed for occasions when instrument ties are impractical.

SUTURE PLACEMENT

There is room for individual preference in the order in which sutures are placed, but it often works well to put the first suture in the middle of the incision and the next two at the $\frac{1}{4}$ and $\frac{3}{4}$ points (figure 2-11). Additional bites are taken to fill in the gaps. When closing irregular lacerations, it is often important to identify landmarks (the vermilion border of the lip, for example) and place sutures at these points before attempting closure of the rest of the wound. Be flexible, think ahead, and do not be reluctant to remove a stitch if it proves to be less than perfect.

Each loop of suture should be deeper than it is wide and wider at its deep end than at its surface (figure 2-12). The spacing between sutures should be slightly less than the distance between the entry and exit points for each individual suture.

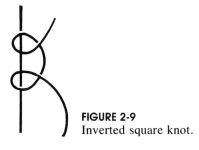

FIGURE 2-9
Inverted square knot.

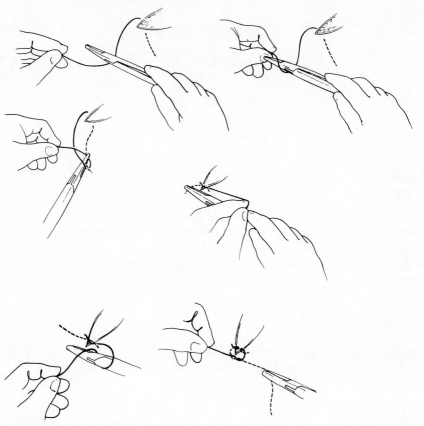

FIGURE 2-10
Instrument tie.

Simple interrupted sutures are used more than all other types combined. They permit careful individual placement of each stitch with the
appropriate degree of tightness. If one stitch breaks or comes untied, the
others are not affected (figure 2-13).

Buried sutures are almost always made of absorbable materials. Take
your tissue bites in the reverse order so that the knot will be on the bottom
of the loop, at some distance from the skin (figure 2-14). Since it's
important to have as little buried suture material as possible, tie a proper
square knot (not a surgeon's knot) and cut the suture ends very short.

Vertical mattress sutures are useful in preventing wound edges from
curling inward and overlapping; this can be a serious problem in areas
where the skin is thin and flexible, such as the back of the hand. They are
also useful in situations where one needs to obliterate subcutaneous dead
space but doesn't want to use buried sutures because of the high risk of

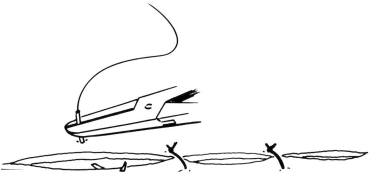

FIGURE 2-11
Closure of wound by fractions.

infection. Alternating vertical mattress and simple interrupted sutures work well in some situations.

The first step in placing a vertical mattress suture is to take just a tiny bite of epidermis on each side of the incision (figure 2-15). Then place the needle backward in your needle holder, lift up on the two ends of the stitch you have just placed, and make a deeper pass with the needle in the opposite direction. Tie the ends in the usual way.

Horizontal mattress sutures are of limited value, being used chiefly to close short skin defects where doing the job quickly is more important than getting a good cosmetic result (figure 2-16).

Corner stitches are used at the apex of V- or Y-shaped incisions where it is important to minimize interference with the blood supply of the acutely angled flap. The suture material passes horizontally through the latter as shown in figure 2-17.

Subcuticular sutures are used (1) in circumstances where not having to

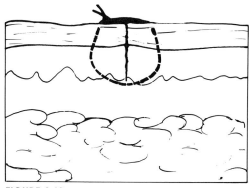

FIGURE 2-12
Profile of completed skin suture.

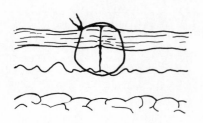
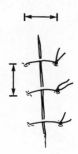

FIGURE 2-13
Simple uninterrupted sutures.

remove the stitches is important (combative children, for example) (2) or on intertriginous areas where wetness is common and it's desirable not to have stitch holes that could serve as portals of infection. This method is not suitable where optimum cosmetic result is expected or where wound separation would be a major complication. Absorbable suture materials are employed. All needle bites are made horizontally into the skin edges.

The sequence is shown in detail in figure 2-18. Start a subcuticular suture by passing the needle horizontally through each skin edge, creating a loop which is then tied carefully (if it should come untied, the incision could fall apart). Then take bites of tissue alternately on the two sides, overlapping slightly so that the lines of tension will be parallel when the incision is pulled closed. Create a loop for tying at the end, and make your last bite in the reverse direction. Tie a square knot, and cut the suture ends right at the knot.

Running sutures can be of three types: plain, locked, or vertical mattress. They are quicker to place than interrupted sutures and are used mostly on surgical incisions which are straight and free of significant tension. They have the following disadvantages: They must be inserted in order from one end of the incision to the other, which would be impractical in irregular wounds. You can't remove just one stitch as might

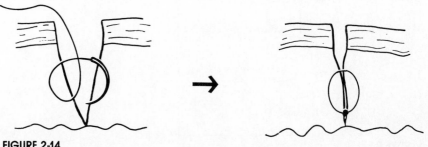

FIGURE 2-14
Buried suture.

(Stage 1)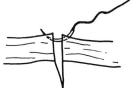

(Stage 2)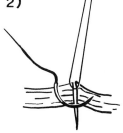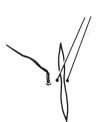

(Stage 3)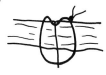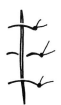

FIGURE 2-15
Vertical mattress sutures.

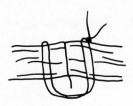

FIGURE 2-16
Horizontal mattress suture.

be indicated if localized infection occurs. If a knot comes untied or the suture breaks, the entire wound loses its support.

The method of placing running sutures is shown in figure 2-19. As with subcuticular sutures, a loop is formed before the last bite, which is taken in the reverse direction. The loop and standing part of the suture are then tied.

Pull-out stitches aren't actually sutures but rather loops of thread placed to facilitate suture removal. They are most useful in situations where edema or poor patient cooperation is likely to make the procedure difficult. Hold a needle backward in your needle holder so that its blunt end passes under each completed suture in turn. Tie the ends to make a loop which can be retrieved and lifted up to make cutting the sutures easier (figure 2-20).

PREPARATION OF INTACT SKIN

Skin should be made as free of bacteria and debris as possible before surgery but not in a way that leaves the epidermis irritated, abraded, or otherwise susceptible to infection. This objective may be achieved by cleaning the area with gauze squares soaked in a detergent-antibacterial solution. The gauze and detergent facilitate mechanical removal of debris

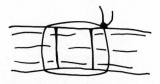
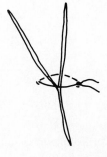

FIGURE 2-17
Corner stitch.

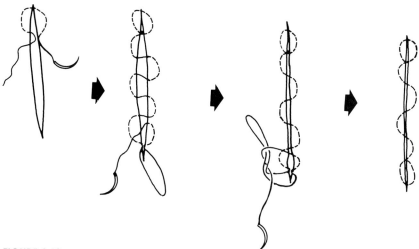

FIGURE 2-18
Subcuticular sutures.

that might harbor bacteria or get into the wound without irritating the skin. Antibacterial agents decrease the bacterial flora significantly but do not kill all the microbes in hair follicles or cutaneous glands. Merely applying a solution to the skin is not sufficient because it does not remove debris which may get into the wound or harbor pathogenic bacteria.

Povidone-iodine preparations (Betadine, other brands) contain the bactericidal agent iodine in low concentrations that are effective but relatively nonirritating. They are available as straight solutions or in combination with a detergent. The latter is preferable for the preparation of intact skin, although the available concentration of iodine is lower than

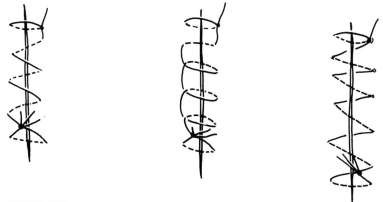

FIGURE 2-19
Plain, locked, and vertical mattress running sutures.

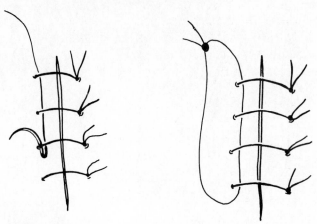

FIGURE 2-20
Pull-out stitch.

with the straight solution. These products should be diluted well with water before use.

Povidone-iodine may cause untoward reactions in patients sensitive to iodine. The iodine is absorbed from raw surfaces and the vaginal mucosa and may cause measurable changes in thyroid function. Two additional unanticipated effects of povidone-iodine have been reported: It may cause a false positive chemical test for blood in the stool or urine. Also, some patients have developed skin irritation when povidone-iodine and Compound Tincture of Benzoin were applied to the same area. This problem may be avoided by rinsing off povidone-iodine before benzoin is applied or by letting benzoin preparations dry completely before the antiseptic is applied.

Chlorhexidine gluconate preparations (Hibiclens) have come on the market more recently than povidone-iodine and are less time-tested. The newer agent has shown superiority in some experimental studies, although the differences do not seem to be of great importance in office practice.

The hands of the person doing the skin preparation should not contaminate the surgical field. For small, low-risk procedures it may be sufficient to wash one's hands before starting. In most cases, however, one should wear gloves or use long dressing forceps to hold the sponges. Always prepare a wider field than you may think will be needed. Drapes slip, wounds turn out to be more extensive than anticipated, and incisions must at times be made larger than originally planned. The prepared area should extend a minimum of 3 inches in all directions from the incision site and a greater distance in many cases. Preparation of surgical sites on an extremity should, in most cases, go all the way around the member.

These preparations are relatively nonirritating but one should be careful that they do not remain in contact with the skin for extended periods of time. For example, if a procedure is being done on a patient's axilla, be sure that some of the cleansing solution does not flow under the patient's shoulder and pool there unrecognized.

Shaving of hair about the surgical site has been largely discontinued because it may abrade the skin and predispose to infection. The benefits of shaving are outweighed by the risk of reduced resistance to infection in the damaged epidermis. Clip the hair with scissors if there is a risk that it will get into the wound and interfere with healing. Do not shave or clip eyebrows; the hair may fail to grow back in these areas, with adverse medicolegal consequences.

PREPARATION OF WOUNDS

An antimicrobial-detergent preparation is used as described above to prepare the skin surrounding a laceration. Reasonable precautions should be taken to keep the agent out of the wound itself to minimize chemical trauma to the tissues. Cleansing procedures within the wound will depend on its nature, location, and level of contamination. A simple incised wound caused by a kitchen knife or piece of broken glass may require nothing more than brief irrigation using a gauze sponge soaked with tap water. Use sterile normal saline solution for more extensive wounds. This can be poured into a sterile basin and applied with a syringe while using a gauze sponge in the other hand to open recesses in the wound and to remove debris mechanically. In some instances one may take an ordinary disposable hypodermic syringe and needle, perhaps a 12-cc syringe with a 20-gauge needle, and use it as a "squirt gun." If a large volume of irrigating fluid is required, hang up a bottle of sterile normal saline solution and let it run into the wound through intravenous tubing.

The use of povidone-iodine solutions for wound irrigation has been advocated without substantial evidence for benefit. The solution is relatively bland, but it has been shown experimentally to interfere with normal healing. Each new generation of surgeons must learn the lesson that an agent which is strong enough to kill pathogens in tissue is also strong enough to damage the tissue itself. If one feels obliged to use povidone-iodine for this purpose, be sure to use only the straight solution without detergents and to dilute it down so that the concentration of the active ingredient does not exceed 1%. If the wound contains debris, as for instance bits of gravel after a fall on a gravel path, it will be necessary to spend time picking out all visible contamination, irrigating the recesses of the wound, and debriding devitalized tissue. Inject a local anesthetic agent before starting major irrigation or debridement. If the skin margins have been contused, they should be excised unless the injury is on the patient's hand or foot. The technique for doing this is discussed in the section on lacerations in Chapter 4.

ANESTHESIA

Anesthesia for most ambulatory surgical procedures is obtained by local injection of an anesthetic solution. The application of intense cold in the form of ethyl chloride spray or a proprietary topical freezing spray may be appropriate for brief procedures, such as the incision of abscesses; this is safer than injecting drugs into hyperemic, possibly infected tissues. Topical application of anesthetic solutions is often effective on the conjunctiva and mucous membranes but seldom for procedures on intact skin; this type of anesthesia is discussed in sections describing specific procedures (in chapters on the eye and nose).

Local anesthesia is usually quite safe if properly done, but life-threatening reactions may occur occasionally. One is obliged to inquire about previous reactions before giving these agents. Careful questioning may be needed to tell whether the patient who reports "allergy" to anesthetic agents is talking about a vasovagal phenomenon, toxicity caused by overdose, simple anxiety, or an allergic reaction. True allergy to lidocaine is quite uncommon. Cross-reactivity between lidocaine and such chemically dissimilar anesthetic agents as procaine, tetracaine, and benzocaine has not been demonstrated.

One must be alert for early evidence of toxicity or allergic reactions. The physician needs to concentrate on the procedure, so the monitoring of pulse, blood pressure, and mental status should be done by a nurse or aide. This personal attention has the additional benefit of helping the patient remain calm and relaxed.

It is often helpful to premedicate a patient before an uncomfortable or anxiety-producing procedure. Short-acting benzodiazepine tranquilizers are helpful for this purpose. They may be taken before the patient leaves home or, if necessary, administered intravenously before the procedure is started. Sedation of this type is practical only if the patient is accompanied by someone who can act as guide and chauffeur.

Injection Anesthesia

Injecting a local anesthetic solution into the tissues induces anesthesia of varying intensity and duration, depending on the agent used, its concentration, and the precision with which it is injected. Lidocaine (Xylocaine, other brands) is deservedly the most popular agent. It is relatively safe,diffuses readily, and goes to work promptly. Its duration of effect is roughly one hour.

Toxic effects appear to be dose-related. They can usually be prevented by limiting the total dose and by aspirating before each infusion to avoid intravascular injection. The manufacturer recommends that the total dose for healthy adults not exceed 300 mg (4.5 mg/kg), or 500 mg (7 mg/kg) if an epinephrine-containing preparation is used. These limits are reduced for children and the elderly. Always use the smallest practical volume of the most dilute solution that will achieve the needed effect.

Preparations of lidocaine with epinephrine 1:200,000 are useful in circumstances where a vasoconstrictive action may reduce capillary bleeding and prolong the duration of anesthetic effect somewhat. However, this same vasoconstrictive effect makes the epinephrine-containing solutions dangerous and therefore contraindicated on the fingers, toes, ears, and penis. Epinephrine should also be avoided in patients with significant cardiovascular disease and those taking a variety of drugs; the manufacturer's literature should be consulted before using this or any local anesthetic agent.

The 1.0% solution, with or without epinephrine, is suitable for infiltration anesthesia. The maximum dose with epinephrine is 50 ml for healthy adults, although it is uncommon to need that much in office surgery. The 0.5% solution is almost as effective and is preferred where large volumes of solution will be needed. Other concentrations are available but seldom needed in primary care.

Mepivacaine (Carbocaine) is a suitable alternative agent, although it is not available with epinephrine. Its effect is slightly longer than that of lidocaine. Bupivacaine (Marcaine, Sensorcaine) 0.25% solution may be kept on hand for the occasional patient who needs a significantly longer-acting local anesthetic drug. Its effects last two to three times as long as lidocaine but are otherwise similar to those of lidocaine and mepivacaine.

Ordinary disposable hypodermic syringes and needles are satisfactory for infiltration anesthesia for the removal of small skin lesions and the repair of small lacerations. Some physicians prefer to use syringes with rings for the thumb, index, and middle fingers; these make it easier to pull back on the plunger to be sure the tip of the needle is not in a blood vessel.

A relatively large needle (perhaps 20 gauge) may be used to withdraw the anesthetic solution from its vial. The actual injection is done with a smaller needle. A 25-gauge needle is easy to use and permits rapid injection, whereas a 27-gauge needle requires more skill and patience but is significantly more comfortable for the patient. Longer needles permit more tissue to be anesthetized with a single skin stick than shorter ones.

In most situations sterile preparation of the skin is done before the anesthetic agent is injected. In selected circumstances, as for example with an extensive injury where the cleansing procedure may be painful, one may elect to do some preliminary preparation, inject the local anesthetic, and then proceed to more vigorous washing.

The procedure for withdrawing the solution from the vial is simple but should be followed with care. The nurse starts by reading the label and then showing it to the physician so that both are absolutely sure that the correct product is being used. The nurse cleans the rubber top of the vial with an antiseptic swab and then holds it in an inverted position to permit withdrawal of the solution. The physician pulls the plunger of the syringe back to fill it with air equivalent in volume to the liquid to be removed, and passes the needle through the rubber stopper (the nurse can help at this point by bumping the bottom of the vial with the heel of one hand, to drive it down over the needle). The physician pushes the plunger to inject air into the vial and pulls back to fill the syringe.

If it appears likely that the syringe will have to be refilled later, the physician detaches the needle from the syringe at this point, leaving it stuck in the rubber cap. Subsequent withdrawals are made without injecting air into the vial to reduce the risk of contamination. These solutions are inexpensive; it is always wiser to discard part of a vial at the end of a procedure than to run a risk of possibly infecting a subsequent patient.

A smaller needle is attached to the syringe and the injection commences. For patient comfort it should be planned to minimize the number of times the skin is penetrated. The actual technique will vary with the nature of the clinical problem. For example, if a skin tumor is to be removed, determine the direction and length of the incision before injecting. Start at one end of the planned incision and inject subcutaneously, advancing the needle 5 mm or so before each bolus. Aspirate for blood before each incremental injection and move the needle tip if any appears in the syringe. Injecting solution into the tumor itself would distort its architecture and interfere with microscopic examination, so avoid this. If more profound anesthesia is desired, a series of intradermal injections may be made along the course of the planned incision after the solution injected subcutaneously has had a few minutes to take effect.

Anesthetic injections for the repair of lacerations can be made through the wound into the subcutaneous tissues. This will cause less discomfort than injecting through the skin.

Digital block is often more satisfactory than direct injection of fingers or toes, especially if the problem involves their distal segments. In actual practice it is better to make a ring block than to attempt precise injection of the digital nerves. This can usually be done by sticking the skin just twice, as shown in figure 2-21. Avoid injecting through the thick palmar or plantar skin. With care a very satisfactory digital block can almost always be achieved with 2 to 3 ml of 1% lidocaine solution (without epinephrine, of course). Onset of anesthesia will take about fifteen minutes.

Always test the anesthetic effect with a needle tip or other sharp object before starting to operate. In many cases the patient will be unable to feel a pinprick but may retain other sensory modalities. It's often wise to tell the patient that he or she may be aware of being worked on, even though pain sensation is blocked.

The onset of a toxic reaction to lidocaine or a similar agent may be heralded by restlessness and anxiety. One may be tempted to inject more anesthetic solution in an effort to reduce the patient's perception of pain, but this will only make the problem worse. It is important to keep the possibility of such toxicity in mind and to stop administration of the drug if its occurrence is suspected.

These reactions involve primarily the central nervous and cardiovascular systems. They may be heralded by restlessness, anxiety, and confusion. Alternatively, the patient may become drowsy or unconscious. Convulsions and respiratory arrest may follow. The cardiovascular effects may start as hypotension and/or bradycardia, possibly followed by arrythmias and cardiac arrest. Initial treatment may include oxygenation, respiratory support, and reassurance to the patient. Intravenous anticonvulsant agents may be tried for persistent convulsions. Intravenous fluids and vasopressors may be needed if cardiovascular function is severely compromised.

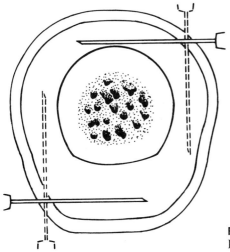

FIGURE 2-21
Digital block.

Cold Anesthesia

Partial anesthesia for brief painful procedures can be obtained by the application of intense cold. If one wishes to snip off a simple skin tag, the area can be numbed by holding the corner of an ice cube against it for a minute or two and then quickly removing the lesion with scissors (using sterile procedure). More profound momentary anesthesia of larger areas can be achieved by spraying ethyl chloride or one of the proprietary freezing sprays onto the skin until the area is covered with frost. The patient will experience some aching as the tissues become cold. Ethyl chloride is highly flammable and must not be used where any degree of fire hazard exists. Cold anesthesia doesn't last more than a few minutes, so preparations for the procedure should be completed before anesthesia is started and the operation should be done quickly.

Simple removal of ingrown toenails can be accomplished with spray anesthesia if the operator is prepared to carry out the procedure quickly. This does not apply to procedures where any cutting or suturing will be done.

Cold is often used for anesthesia in situations where injection of anesthetic solutions is contraindicated because of the presence of infection, most commonly for incision and drainage of abscesses. There is difference of opinion on this point: Some have injected lidocaine solutions into the tissue overlying an abscess with apparent impunity, but others believe it safer to spray ethyl chloride or one of the proprietary freezing sprays onto the site of the planned incision. Either way, it is important to remember that skin anesthesia will not affect the deeper reaches of an abscess. The subcutaneous tissues are much less sensitive than skin, but one should be as gentle to them as is consistent with adequate drainage of the lesion.

IMMOBILIZATION OF CHILDREN

The first step in immobilizing a child for a procedure is, quite simply, to try to make immobilization unnecessary by gaining the child's confidence and cooperation. Patients under 4 years of age cannot be expected to respond to verbal explanations beyond simple reassurance that everything is "OK," but they are very sensitive to nonverbal cues from their parents and from medical personnel. Therefore the first step is to deal with the parents' feelings. If necessary, sit down with them for a few minutes of reassurance and explanation. Move slowly in the child's presence, speak calmly and in a low voice, and avoid words like "hurt" and "shot." Set up completely for the procedure before bringing the child into the room. Never lie to a child about what is going to happen, and try to discourage parents from doing so. Fear and resistance are to be expected in some children despite the best of preparation, though, so at some point you usually must make a decision to immobilize the child and get the procedure over with as quickly as practical. Use a papoose board (figure 2-22) or a folded sheet (figure 2-23). Have enough staff people and family members present to keep the child restrained enough that you can complete your procedure promptly and (hopefully) with no lapses of sterile technique. If the head needs to be immobilized, have an attendant sit on a stool at the head of the table with forearms resting on the table and one hand on either side of the patient's head. If an extremity is to be treated, have the attendant "shake hands" with the hand or foot involved. Reward the child with some kind words and some small gift afterward, and his or her anger won't last long.

The older the child, the more cooperation you can gain by talking directly with the patient. Explain your plans in simple terms, let the child know that there will be some discomfort, and give reassurance that you will be as gentle as possible. Distract the youngster during the procedure by asking about schoolwork, hobbies, or whatever else interests the patient.

The decision to let family members stay in the room should be made on an individual basis, often with the patient and parents participating in the choice. If a parent wants to leave, by all means encourage that decision;

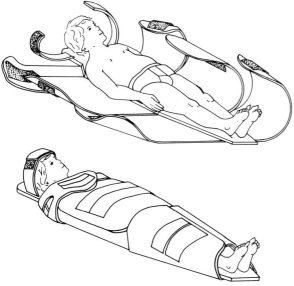

FIGURE 2-22
Immobilizing a child with a papoose board.

an adult who vomits or faints during a pediatric procedure can create major problems. If the adult is unduly anxious or if there is a relationship of clinging mutual dependency between parent and child, it may be necessary to separate the two.

TETANUS IMMUNIZATION

Appropriate decisions about tetanus immunization require accurate information about previous injections. This may often be obtained from the physician's clinical notes or an immunization record maintained by the family. Dependable inferences can sometimes be derived from other historical data, as for example if the patient has been in the armed forces or a child has been under regular supervision by another physician known to follow proper preventive care procedures. One is often faced with ambiguous situations in which the interval since the last booster can only be guessed at. The cost and risk of tetanus immunization are minor compared to the ravages of the disease, so it is always preferable to err on the side of giving injections that might not be necessary.

Active immunization is obtained through the use of adsorbed tetanus toxoid. For children under age 7 it is routinely given in a combined product with diphtheria toxoid and pertussis vaccine (called DTP). There is a pediatric product containing no pertussis antigen (DT) for limited indications. The product used for adults and children age 7 or older contains tetanus toxoid with a reduced dose of diphtheria toxoid (Td). Straight tetanus toxoid is also available. Td is the preferred product for booster injections at the time of injury; it provides supplemental protection for two potentially devastating diseases at essentially the same cost and risk as protection against tetanus alone. The standard dose for all of these preparations is 0.5 ml intramuscularly.

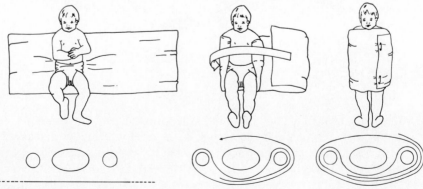

FIGURE 2-23
Immobilizing a child with a folded sheet.

Passive immunization is provided by tetanus immune globulin (TIG), available in single-dose vials of 250 units. Patients who say they are "allergic to tetanus" are usually talking about adverse reactions to tetanus antitoxin, an obsolete product derived from horse serum. These patients can and should receive Td and TIG.

Most children in the United States have received adequate immunization against tetanus by the time they enter school. The highest incidence of clinical tetanus in this country today is among older people, some of whom were never immunized and many of whom have not received decennial boosters. Many of these cases occur in patients with trivial wounds or in whom no recognized wound has occurred, emphasizing the importance of this very simple but effective immunization procedure.

A clean incised wound sustained within a building carries little risk of tetanus. However, the occasion when such an injury is being treated is a convenient time to check on the patient's immunization status and give a booster if it isn't certain that this has been done within the past decade (the term *booster* is variously defined; it is used here to signify a supplemental dose of an immunizing agent, without reference to the reason for giving it).

A puncture wound or a laceration involving devitalized tissue is more tetanus-prone. An injury sustained in proximity to earth, especially one in a barnyard situation, carries greatly increased risk of the disease. Previously immunized patients with these types of wounds should receive tetanus toxoid if they have not received boosters in recent years; recommendations from different sources give different cut-off intervals, but five years seems reasonable. Tetanus immune globulin should also be given if there is a possibility that more than ten years have elapsed since the last toxoid injection.

Persons who have not been immunized against tetanus previously should receive both Td and TIG injections, and arrangements should be made for subsequent Td doses. The second shot should be given four to eight weeks after the first, the third six to twelve months after the second, and subsequent doses at ten-year intervals.

ANTIBIOTICS

It is not often necessary or desirable to prescribe antibiotics after office surgical procedures. The physician who prescribes them usually sees patients heal promptly. The doctor who uses careful technique and avoids antibiotics sees equally favorable outcomes. The decision to use antibiotics will vary with the nature of the lesion, its location on the body, and the general health of the patient. For example, a human bite involving the extensor tendon sheaths of the hand of an alcoholic patient would call for antimicrobial treatment, while a clean incised wound on the scalp of a healthy child would not. Whenever possible, start the antibiotics before performing a procedure that carries a significant risk of infection. Stop them no more than two or three days later to minimize interference with the body's normal bacterial flora unless there is evidence of active infection.

DRESSINGS

Wound dressings serve many objectives which vary from one patient to another. They provide protection from contamination with dirt, irritants, and pathogenic microorganisms. They absorb blood and other exudates. They immobilize injured parts, either through the stiffness of the materials or by means of splints incorporated in the dressings. In some situations they are employed to apply medications to the skin. They can be used to compress the underlying tissues to obliterate dead space and control edema. Dressings may give comfort by protecting tender areas and by concealing unsightly lesions from the view of the patient and other people. Their use may also prevent meddlesome interventions by patients or families who do not understand that wounds heal best when left alone.

Dressings should have a neat and professional appearance since their appearance may take on major importance to patients and families. It's important that they remain functional until it is time for them to come off; healing may be greatly impaired if dressings which look good initially slip out of place, permit wound contamination, or otherwise fail to accomplish their purposes.

Many excellent dressing products are available from commercial suppliers. The suggestions made herein are not intended to be exhaustive; brand names are mentioned for illustration only. Each practice should make its own choices based on the patient problems likely to be encountered. There is room for the expression of personal preferences and ingenuity.

In the paragraphs that follow all the components that may be incorporated in a dressing are listed in order from the skin to the outside. Most dressings will include only a few of these elements; the reader can select those applicable to each patient's needs.

Some *skin preparation* may be indicated before the dressing is applied. If dried blood is present, it should be rinsed off with sterile water or saline or, if one prefers, hydrogen peroxide solution; this is done primarily for aesthetic reasons. If adherence of the dressing is likely to be a problem, because of oiliness or perspiration, you may want to apply tincture of benzoin, either as a liquid or in a proprietary spray, to enhance the adherence of adhesive tape. Benzoin is somewhat unpleasant to use; it discolors objects it touches and leaves a sticky feeling on the hands of people who work with it. However, it is readily removed with alcohol or other organic solvents. For maximum adherence apply adhesive tape after the benzoin has become sticky to touch but before it has dried completely. One caution: Tincture of benzoin and povidone-iodine antiseptic products have been reported to interact in a way that may cause skin burns. The latter should be washed off before benzoin is applied to the same area. A proprietary liquid called Mastisol is preferred by some physicians for many of the same indications.

The use of *drains* is discussed in the section on abscesses. The topical use of *medications* is described in appropriate sections.

Small *sterile adhesive strips* (Steri-strips, other brands) may be used in place of sutures to close small wounds. They are useful on irregular finger wounds where preservation of tissue is important, provided that the skin is dry when they are applied and that the digit is immobilized with a splint for a few days. They can also be employed to reinforce healing incisions when sutures are removed early, before healing has progressed to substantial strength.

If it appears likely that the dressing will tend to stick to the skin or sutures one should consider inserting an *antistick product* such as Telfa or Adaptic between the skin and the absorbent layer of the dressing. The only significant drawback to its use is a tendency to trap moisture. This is usually not a practical problem in the management of closed lacerations and excised skin lesions if just a single thickness of the material is used and if other layers of the dressing facilitate absorption and diffusion of moisture. Antibiotic ointments can accomplish the same objective but with greater risk of maceration and allergic reactions.

Bulk in the form of gauze squares, fluffs, or rolled products such as Kerlix will absorb exudate and protect wounds from external contamination. Enough thickness should be provided so that exudates do not reach the top of the dressing, creating a moist track along which pathogens can migrate down to the skin. Aluminum *splints* of various types may be incorporated in dressings, most often for finger lesions, to immobilize the digit and to protect against bumping the part in the course of daily activities. Their use should be discontinued after no more than seven days because of the risk of loss of joint mobility. Temporary fixation of larger joints, most commonly the knee, can be achieved by incorporating long plaster splints into dressings.

Compression bandages are used to minimize dead space and to control local edema and venous stasis. They can also help to discourage bleeding into or from the wound but should not be used for this purpose to the exclusion of other, more reliable forms of hemostasis. The traditional rubber-thread elastic bandage, often called by the brand name Ace, provides good, even compression when skillfully applied. Cotton elastic bandages are less expensive but provide less even compression. Both these types tend to slide out of position easily; when this happens, some areas may be inadequately covered, while others may be compressed severely enough to compromise local circulation. These problems may be minimized by using a self-adherent elastic bandage such as Coban, although it is important that this product be applied with less tension than standard elastic bandages since it does not "sag" significantly with time.

The ability to apply elastic bandages properly, especially to irregular areas like the hand and foot, comes only with practice. Always unroll the bandage in its natural direction, avoiding excessive tension. Learn to plan ahead and follow the contours of the extremity, turning the course of the bandage only slightly so that the compression will not be excessive on one side. The following procedure may be used to wrap a foot and ankle: Start by taking a turn around the ankle. Then unroll toward the foot, covering it with two or three turns down to the base of the toes before working back toward the ankle. Try to cover the malleoli of the ankles as you follow a modified figure eight pattern: one or two turns around the ankle, then two or three turns around the foot, then repeat the pattern. If the purpose of the dressing requires coverage of the leg above the ankle, remember that any dressing applied to a conical part of the body (such as the middle third of the leg) will tend to slip distally with the patient's normal motions. Either carry the bandaging up over the largest part of the calf almost to the knee, or if this is impractical, use adhesive tape to anchor the top of the circumferential dressing.

The top layer of a dressing serves to hold all the others in place. A compression dressing, if applied, may serve this purpose. A physician with imagination can find ways to use short lengths of a self-adherent product like Coban to make effective, unobtrusive dressings for irregular areas such as the hand. Nonelastic self-adherent gauze products such as Kling are available in various widths. Physicians who see large numbers of work-related injuries often prefer to use knitted tubular-gauze products such as Tubegauz and Flexknit; these also are marketed in a variety of sizes.

Circumferential dressings of the fingers, arms, and legs tend to slide distally because of the somewhat conical shape of the areas to which they are applied. Finger dressings can be anchored in place either with adhesive tape or by carrying the dressing up around the wrist. Tape may also be used at the top and bottom of arm and leg dressings. In all these areas it is important not to apply tape all the way around since this could lead to a tourniquet effect. Leave a gap of a centimeter or two between the ends of the tape.

It is important that a circumferential dressing be applied in a way that minimizes edema and will not constrict the extremity unduly if local tissue swelling occurs. If compression is not needed, the dressing may be applied only to the affected segment if there is no significant tension and the dressing is loose enough that local swelling can occur without causing a tourniquet effect. If compression is utilized, the dressing should be no tighter than needed, and in most cases it should be continued distally to the base of the toes or fingers. Whenever a circumferential dressing is applied, the patient or family should be instructed to consult the physician promptly if unexpected swelling, skin discoloration, or pain occurs.

Adhesive tapes are available in many sizes and materials. Paper tapes adhere well, permit moisture to evaporate from the skin, and are strong enough for most uses. The newer cloth tapes are excellent for applications such as ankle strapping where tensile strength is important. The traditional zinc oxide and cloth type adheres less well than the newer products and occasionally causes severe local reactions. Two errors in the use of adhesive tapes are commonly seen. One is failure to use enough of it; the tape should extend far enough from the rest of the dressing that the tension on it runs essentially parallel to the skin surface ("in shear"). The other error is to apply tape to skin that is moist, oily, or contaminated with other substances (talc, for example) that interfere with adhesion.

Small ready-to-use dressings, commonly called by the brand name Band-Aids, are available in many sizes and shapes. Some come in special shapes for special applications, such as fingertip dressings. The standard small sizes have numerous uses in a medical office, such as covering injection sites and treating small cuts sustained by staff members. These products tend to trap moisture, however, and should not be worn long enough to cause maceration of the underlying skin.

Flexible collodion solution or a proprietary occlusive spray such as Aeroplast, both of which leave a plastic film when they dry, can substitute for dressings in some circumstances. For example, scalp lacerations are difficult to dress, have a favorable prognosis, and heal well when covered with nothing more than a film of plastic.

Some lesions require no dressing at all, other than the one provided by the normal healing process (we call it a scab). With many such lesions it is permissible for the patient to wash the area, but prolonged wetness and maceration must be avoided. Lacerations in locations unlikely to be traumatized and which are healing normally a few days after primary closure fit this category. Lesions around the mouth are left open since dressings would become contaminated quickly. The same consideration applies to most lesions about the perineum.

A number of special considerations apply to dressings for lesions of the hands and fingers. Immobilization may be very important if tendon sheaths are involved, if there is risk of infection, or in other high-risk situations. If an injury may heal with residual limitation of finger motion, it is essential that it be immobilized in the position of function, with all joints slightly flexed (figure 2-24). Children too young to understand the

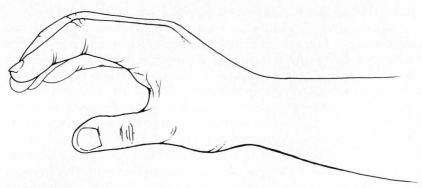

FIGURE 2-24
Position of function.

importance of leaving dressings undisturbed may try to remove them. If circulation is impaired, it may be important to leave fingertips out of a dressing so they can be watched. Elevation of the injured part will minimize local swelling and discomfort. Loss of the use of a hand, especially the dominant one, may be quite disabling; immobilization of one hand impairs the ability to carry on many activities of daily living, including washing of the other hand. A patient whose work is inherently dirty may find it difficult to earn a living without soiling a hand dressing so much that daily (or more frequent) changes are necessary.

To illustrate the utilization of these principles, let us assume that a 3-year-old child has sustained a crush injury of the ulnar side of one hand. After examination, x-rays, and repair of the laceration, a dressing is applied as follows: A piece of fine-mesh gauze saturated with petrolatum is applied to keep the dressing from sticking to the wound. A few layers of gauze squares are applied over the injured area, and smaller pieces are placed between the fingers. A wad of gauze fluffs is placed next to the palm and fingers to hold the hand in the position of function. A self-adherent elastic bandage is now applied with only minimum tension, leaving the fingertips and the thumb free. It is continued almost to the wrist joint, permitting wrist motion but keeping the dressing from sliding distally. The last turn of the dressing ends on the ulnar side of the hand where the child will be least likely to find it and start unwrapping the dressing (figure 2-25). A sling may be provided to keep the hand from hanging down.

The longer the interval between dressing changes, the less chance of disrupting the healing process or introducing infection. A dressing may need to be removed when it is saturated with exudate, when a drain needs to come out, if unexplained pain or fever occurs, if the outside becomes unsightly, when it is time to remove sutures, or when healing has progressed to a point where the dressing is no longer needed. Dressings can often be removed from cleanly incised wounds two or three days after they have been sutured, unless contamination is likely to be a problem or immobilization of the part is still indicated. Dermicel or other porous adhesive tape can be applied to the incision to minimize irritation and pulling on the sutures.

Opinions differ with regard to the desirability of having patients or families change dressings at home. In some instances this may be necessary because of considerations of distance or economics. However, few family members are prepared to follow aseptic procedure faithfully, and it seems likely that most closed lesions will heal about as well with no dressing at all as with one applied under the usual home conditions.

SUTURE REMOVAL

Sutures on the face and scalp may be removed in three days and should be out by the fifth day to prevent punctate scars (stitch marks) from forming. Since small children may be fearful of suture removal procedures, you may elect to close scalp wounds with polyglycolate or chromic gut stitches which will dissolve out by themselves; for ideal cosmetic results don't use this method on the face. Sutures elsewhere on the body should come out after seven to ten days, or longer if the local circulation is compromised.

Scissors for removing stitches should have fine points that can slide easily under sutures. Specially designed stitch removal scissors are available, or one can use straight fine point scissors of a type designed for eye surgery. Small hemostats or thumb forceps with small serrations are

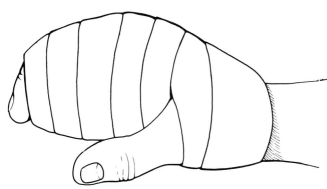

FIGURE 2-25
Functional hand dressing.

used to grasp the suture material; toothed tissue forceps are unsatisfactory for this purpose.

If there is a dressing on the wound when sutures are to be removed, no special skin preparation is needed unless there is some clotted blood present which needs to be washed away. If the patient presented for removal with no dressing, simple washing with soap and water will minimize the chance of introducing infection during the procedure. Avoid harsh detergents or bactericidal agents, though, to obviate the risk of their being introduced into the tissues as the stitches are pulled through.

To remove a simple interrupted suture, grasp one of the short ends just above the knot, raise the knot a millimeter or so, and cut the suture with scissors just below the knot. This technique minimizes the amount of contaminated suture material which must be pulled through the subcutaneous tissues in the removal process. If the sutures are being removed early for cosmetic reasons it's often wise to minimize tension on the skin edges for a few days by applying sterile adhesive strips.

Further dressings may not be necessary if the wound has closed primarily, although the risk of infection seeding through the stitch holes can be reduced by keeping a dry dressing in place for a few hours after the procedure.

SUGGESTED READING

Clavin HD: Practical tips for office surgery: Commonsense advice from a plastic surgeon. *Postgrad Med* 74(2):303, 1983.

Epstein E, Epstein E Jr: *Skin Surgery,* 5th ed. Springfield, Ill., Charles C Thomas, 1982.

Riley WB: Wound healing. *Amer Fam Phys* 24(5):107, 1981.

Rodeheaver G, Bellamy W, Kody M, Spatafora G, Fitten L, Leyden K, Edlich R: Bactericidal activity and toxicity of iodine-containing solutions in wounds. *Arch Surg* 117:181, 1982.

Schultz BD, Mckinney P: *Office Practice of Skin Surgery.* Philadelphia, Saunders, 1985.

Sebben JE: Surgical antiseptics. *J Amer Acad Dermatol* 9:759, 1983.

chapter 3

Nontraumatic Skin and Subcutaneous Lesions

Consultant: RICHARD S. MORAITES, M.D.

Patients with relatively straightforward surgical problems suitable for office management are seen frequently in family practice. It is a convenience for both physicians and patients to be able to treat them promptly and effectively without referring them out. The excision of a small skin tumor will be described completely to illustrate a number of fine points in nontraumatic office surgery. Other procedures will be discussed in less detail.

EXCISION OF SKIN TUMORS

A hypothetical patient presents a solitary 1-cm tumor of uncertain etiology on the forearm. Its appearance does not suggest melanoma or other malignancy. You recommend removal, both for diagnosis and (hopefully) for cure, and the patient gives consent.

The patient removes any clothing that might become stained by blood or skin-cleaning agents and lies on the examining-treatment table with the arm lying out on an arm board. You plan a bay leaf shaped incision considering the size and shape of the lesion, the natural lines of the skin, and the need to pull the wound together for closure after removal of the mass.

Local anesthesia may be administered either before or after skin preparation. The sterile technique will be simpler if you elect to do the injection first. An excellent agent for such a procedure (not involving a digit) is 0.5% lidocaine with epinephrine. Wipe the rubber stopper of the vial with a disposable alcohol swab. Use a disposable 3-ml hypodermic syringe with a 20-gauge needle. Pull the plunger back to admit 2 to 3 ml of air. Enter the vial with the needle, inject the air, and withdraw an equal volume of anesthetic solution. Change to a 27-gauge, 1-inch needle. Clean the skin surrounding the tumor with the alcohol swab, and inject the agent subcutaneously, covering the area of your planned incision. Plan the injection to minimize the number of times you will need to pierce the skin. Be sure to include the area under the tumor and areas that will be invaded if you need to undermine the skin edges before closure. Pull the plunger back each time before injecting the agent to be sure the needle tip is not in a blood vessel. For the most profound anesthesia, wait a few minutes and then inject small amounts of the agent intradermally along the course of your planned incision.

The next step is skin preparation. If the patient's arm is unusually hairy, you may want to clip any hairs that could get into your surgical field, but shaving is not indicated. Wash the area vigorously with an iodophor or chlorhexidine preparation and gauze sponges, preparing an area at least 3 inches (8 cm) in all directions from the lesion. Don your sterile gloves. Drape the field, using a sterile disposable or cloth draping sheet with a hole in its center ("fenestrated"). Arrange your sterile instruments and supplies for convenient access.

If local anesthesia is not performed until after preparation and draping have been done, an assistant will need to hold the vial firmly in an inverted position while you inject air and withdraw the anesthetic agent with sterile technique (figure 3-1). Either way, touch the injected area lightly with a needle or scalpel tip to be sure it is completely numb before beginning to cut.

If you are not using a disposable scalpel, attach a fresh #15 blade to your scalpel handle; hold the blade with a hemostat to eliminate the risk of cutting your fingers. With the sharp side of the scalpel blade turned upward, use its tip to scratch the patient's skin to mark your intended line of incision. Grasp the scalpel as you would a pen, lay the heel of your hand on the patient's forearm for steadiness, and make your incision, starting at the end farthest from you. Stretch and steady the skin using the thumb and index finger of your opposite hand. Ideally, you should cut through the full thickness of the skin into the softer subcutaneous tissues with a single pass of the scalpel blade. A second or third pass may be necessary at times, but avoid making multiple shallow, irregular cuts that leave jagged skin edges. The skin is more rigid and resistant to cutting than the subcutaneous tissue, making it possible to tell by feel when you have cut through the dermis.

Once the incision is well started, grasp the end of the specimen farthest from you with a tissue forceps to give you better control of the tissues as you finish your incision. Alternatively, place a single suture through the distal tip of the specimen for traction. After the skin is cut completely, lift up the forceps or traction suture and cut the specimen free of the underlying connective tissue. Put it in a bottle containing 10% formalin or other fixative, and be sure the container is labeled immediately.

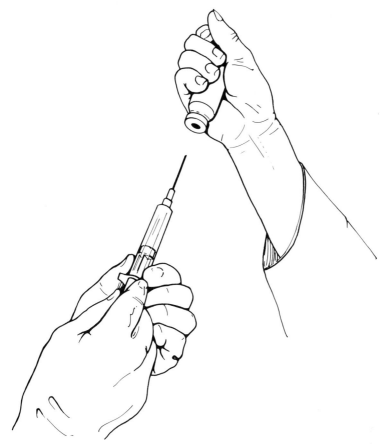

FIGURE 3-1
Obtaining anesthetic agent while gloved.

Hemostasis comes next. Resist the urge to grasp blindly with hemostats; doing so is often unproductive and entails a risk of damaging underlying nerves, tendons, or other structures. Control bleeding for the moment with a gauze sponge held with steady pressure. Many small bleeding points will stop spontaneously if compressed for two minutes or longer. Those that do not may be grasped individually with hemostats as the sponge is gradually removed from the operative field. Do not use a wiping motion with sponges because this abrades tissues and tends to dislodge clots that are forming in the open ends of small vessels in the wound.

Small bleeding vessels may stay closed if a clamp is applied to them for a few minutes and then released. Larger ones, especially arterial "pumpers," will need to be ligated. If you have a gloved assistant, one of you can hold the hemostats up while the other applies ligatures of gut or polyglycolate suture material. If you are working alone it is more practical to use suture-ligatures of the same material. Pass your needle beneath an offending vessel using the hemostat for guidance and support. Tie the first turn of the knot with the instrument in place, and then remove the hemostat. Tighten the knot, and put another turn on top of it to make a square knot. Let the tissues relax into their normal position to be sure the bleeding has stopped. Then cut the suture ends very close to the knot.

The next step is to pull the wound edges together to determine if closure can be obtained without significant tension. If necessary, undermine the skin flaps: Lift up each skin edge in turn and make a cut about 1 cm in width in the subcutaneous space just under and parallel to the skin. Hemostasis can usually be obtained by direct pressure through the undermined skin.

A few buried gut or polyglycolate sutures may be placed to approximate the subcutaneous tissues, but they usually are not needed. Skin closure is obtained with simple interrupted monofilament sutures, most often 5/0 size. A dressing for such a procedure might include an antistick pad (Telfa, Adaptic, etc.), some folded gauze squares, and adhesive tape. The tape should run almost all the way around the extremity, but be sure to leave a gap to prevent a "tourniquet effect," with edema formation distal to the constricted point. The wound should be inspected in two or three days; if it is healing well at that time, you might elect to apply only a large sterile adhesive strip or a piece of "paper" adhesive tape to protect the stitches until they are removed.

INCISIONAL BIOPSY

If the lesion is so large that excising it completely for diagnosis is impractical, a portion of it may be removed for microscopic examination. This can be done in two ways: A sharp-knife excision of an ellipse of tissue or a punch biopsy. With either technique, select a typical-appearing part of the lesion. Some pathologists prefer to have a portion of the adjacent normal skin in the specimen (figure 3-2). The technique for sharp-knife incisional biopsy is similar to that for excision (previous section) except for the location and size of the incision. Undermining of wound edges and control of individual bleeding points are seldom needed. Closure is usually obtained with sterile adhesive strips or one or two simple sutures.

PUNCH BIOPSY

Biopsy specimens can also be obtained easily with reusable or disposable circular biopsy punches. These consist of a sharpened tubular cutting

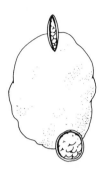 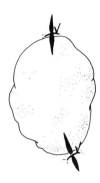

FIGURE 3-2
Sites for incisional biopsy.

blade mounted on a simple handle. To obtain a punch biopsy, select a suitable site as described in the previous section, prepare the skin surface, inject a local anesthetic, and then cut a cylindrical specimen by rotating the instrument. Once you have cut through the skin into the softer subcutaneous tissue, lift the specimen with a skin hook or forceps and cut it free with a scalpel or scissors. Sterile adhesive strips or a simple stitch may be used to close the defect, although this usually isn't necessary with 5-mm or smaller-size punches.

LIGATION OF PEDUNCULATED MASSES

Small pedunculated skin masses are easily removed by tying a string around them tightly enough to cut off their circulation and then letting them drop off spontaneously. The procedure is simple; there is no need for anesthesia, sterile technique, elaborate equipment, or technical expertise. It is suitable only for lesions with slender, well-defined stalks whose circulation can be blocked completely by a simple ligature.

The procedure has certain disadvantages. Tissue is not available for microscopic examination. Some patients may resent paying for a procedure they could have done themselves. The shriveled lesion may persist for a fortnight or more before it falls off. The indications for the maneuver are limited, but it may be indicated in patients who fear anesthetic injections or are allergic to the agents, where cost is an overriding consideration, and where the lesion is clearly not malignant.

A sturdy piece of braided suture material, such as 3/0 polyester, is suggested (monofilament materials don't hold knots as well). Have the patient or an assistant hold the lesion up so that the ligature can be applied to normal skin at its base. Loop the thread around the tissue, make a surgeon's knot (overhand knot with an extra turn), and gradually pull it tight. Advise the patient that a transient stinging sensation may be felt as this is done. Once the knot is tight enough to cut off circulation, apply a square knot over it and cut the ends short. The patient may wash the area normally but should not allow it to be wet for prolonged periods. Mild erythema of the surrounding skin may appear; it does not necessarily signify infection.

EXCISION OF LIPOMA

Removal of benign subcutaneous fatty tumors (lipomas) is an elective matter unless the mass is growing rapidly or has other characteristics that raise the issue of possible malignancy. Many lipomas are treated expectantly because the patient perceives the discomfort of surgery or the resulting scar to be more of a problem than the mass itself. Others are left alone because the patient has so many of them that it would be impractical to excise them all. Patients are most likely to want them removed if they are rubbing on the waistband or bra strap or if they are thought to be unsightly. The decision to excise a lipoma should not be made lightly because some of them are bigger and deeper than they appear and the surgery may turn out to be more extensive than expected.

Explanation to the patient, consent, skin preparation, and draping are carried out in the usual way. A local anesthetic agent is injected into both the incision site and the tissues adjacent to the lipoma. It may be necessary to make supplemental injections as the operation proceeds. Make a straight incision over the mass. Continue your dissection down to the tumor, doing as much of it as practical by the blunt method: Insert the end of a hemostatic forceps into the area you want to enter and spread the tips to force the connective tissue apart. Find a "plane of cleavage" along the surface of the lipoma and dissect it away from the surrounding tissue, working first in one direction and then in another. Once a significant part of the lipoma is exposed, put traction on it, either manually or by means of a traction suture, to make the cleavage planes more evident and accessible. At some points blunt dissection will prove unsuccessful; sturdier tissue bands can be cut with knife or scissors, but grasp them with a hemostat first so they can be ligated easily if they prove to contain small blood vessels. Work slowly and cautiously. Dissect close to the surface of the lipoma itself. Identify adjacent nerves, tendons, or blood vessels, and be careful not to disturb them.

Once the lipoma has been dissected free and preserved for your pathologist to examine, decide what must be done to eliminate the resulting "dead space." In some instances this will require only a few buried sutures. Other cases will require both careful suturing and external compression. Close the skin and dress the wound in the usual manner.

Excisional biopsies of lymph nodes are performed in essentially the same way as removal of lipomas. However, caution is required because these structures are often deeper than they appear from the outside, because they may bleed freely, and because some of them are close to vital structures such as pleura or major nerves.

UNINFECTED SEBACEOUS CYSTS

Sebaceous cysts occur primarily on the head and upper trunk, particularly on the face and neck and about the ears. When not infected, they contain cottage cheese-like sebum. They typically grow very slowly. Some patients describe spontaneous rupture and emptying of their cysts, followed by gradual reaccumulation of their contents. Sebaceous cysts can often be differentiated from lipomas by their location and the fact that they are attached to (indeed, part of) the overlying skin.

To excise a sebaceous cyst, prepare the skin and drape the patient as previously described. Draping, surgical access, and dressings in some locations, such as behind the ears, may tax your ingenuity. Local anesthesia requires care since the lesion is very close to the skin surface. Inject your planned incision site intradermally, and try to infiltrate the agent around (but not in) the cyst. As with lipomas, be prepared to make supplemental injections as the operation proceeds.

Try to determine where the cyst attaches to the skin, and make a bay leaf shaped incision incorporating this area. The length of the incision should about equal the diameter of the cyst. Cut through the epidermis and dermis, but no deeper. Using blunt dissection, shell the lesion out of the surrounding connective tissue, ideally removing the cyst and the overlying ellipse of skin as a single intact specimen. Don't be surprised if the cyst breaks, but do be careful not to leave any sebum in the tissues. Eliminate any significant dead space with absorbable sutures, close the skin, and apply a dressing if practical. Around the ear and nose, dressings may be more trouble than they are worth.

INFECTED SEBACEOUS CYSTS

Patients frequently request treatment for their sebaceous cysts only after infection occurs. The typical history is one of slow appearance of the mass over a period of years, followed by rapidly increasing size and inflammation in just a few days' time. The lesion is typically reddened, warm to touch, firm, and tender. These lesions should be opened under freeze anesthesia. Postpone definitive surgery for at least six weeks because manipulating infected tissue might cause dissemination of bacteria and because the presence of suture material would predispose to local suppuration.

After assembling a scalpel (preferably with #12 blade), hemostat, and dressing materials, wash the area gently and apply a freezing spray until a frost appears on the skin. Incise the cyst quickly and express its contents gently, catching them in sterile gauze pads. Use the hemostat to tease one corner of a gauze square into a wick shape, and insert it into the incision to keep it from closing prematurely. Apply a dressing. Have the patient return in one or at most two days to have the wick removed and a fresh dressing applied. Antibiotics are indicated only in selected cases.

Offer the patient the benefit of definitive excision six weeks or more later, although some lesions will not refill and need not be excised.

SUBCUTANEOUS ABSCESSES

The patient with a typical "boil" may describe a solitary tender mass which appeared in the past few days, or the history may be that of a "crop" of boils appearing sequentially over a period of weeks or months. Sometimes an abscess will undergo spontaneous partial drainage through a small hole which then closes up, permitting the lesion to grow again. This cycle can repeat itself until adequate surgical drainage is accomplished.

As bacteria (most commonly staphylococci) multiply in tissue, they induce an inflammatory response, local necrosis, and unsuccessful attempt at cure by the body's defenses. The purulent mass grows in size and pressure until it breaks and drains. Clinically, there is an early stage when the infection is not sharply localized; attempts to open it at this time will create what can only be described as a "bloody mess." Thus an early abscess which is not sharply defined should not be opened. Prescribe warm applications and an appropriate antibiotic, and recheck the patient in a day or two. After the abscess coalesces, as demonstrated by the appearance of fluctuance and perhaps central softening, drainage will be effective and easily accomplished.

Authorities differ on the desirability of using injection anesthesia for incision and drainage of abscesses. The author is persuaded that the risks of inducing bacteremia and/or intravascular injection of the anesthetic agent are sufficient that local application of intense cold is preferable in most cases. Spray the area with ethyl chloride or other freezing agent until frost appears; this may take longer than you would expect because the area is warm and hyperemic. If freeze anesthesia is impractical, the area can be injected carefully with a small volume of lidocaine with epinephrine, being careful not to inject into a blood vessel or the abscess cavity.

Have the patient remove enough clothing to obviate the risk of soiling. Wash the area without attempting to create sterility. Using a scalpel with a #12 blade, open the abscess widely and boldly: One quick inward stab, pull down and out to complete the cut, and the job is done (figure 3-3). Be prepared to catch the pus with gauze sponges in the other hand. Explore the abscess cavity gently with a hemostat; older authorities speak of breaking up loculations with forceps, but this seems more likely to induce bacteremia than to improve the drainage except in major abscesses of long duration. Gently express whatever pus will come out easily, but don't use force and don't expect to get it all. Irrigation of the abscess cavity is seldom indicated in the primary care setting.

Insert a wick to prevent the incision from closing prematurely. For small abscesses, simply twist the corner of a gauze square into a wick shape and insert it. For larger lesions use Penrose drain material or pieces of rubber glove which have been cut to a dumbell shape. Apply a bulky dressing. Remove the drain in one or at most two days.

The vast majority of abscesses will heal promptly once they have been opened adequately. In the remainder there is almost always a reason for failure to close, such as impaired local circulation or continued fecal contamination from a pararectal abscess-fistula.

Carbuncles are multiple, interconnected abscesses that tend to occur in areas such as the back of the neck, the shoulders, and the buttocks which have thick skin and dense subcutaneous tissue. They tend to burrow and

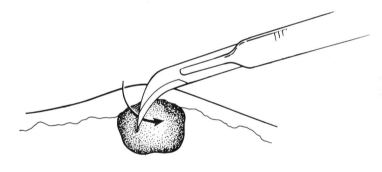

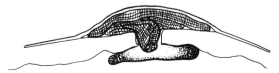

FIGURE 3-3
Incision and drainage of abscess.

become loculated, sometimes with extensive subcutaneous necrosis. Antistaphylococcal antibiotics should be started before surgery is done. A single drainage point is often insufficient; multiple incisions, sometimes in a grid pattern, may be needed. Rest and warm applications are also used.

Abscesses in the pads of the fingers are called *felons*. They, too, may require extensive drainage. A deep incision is made through the side of the distal segment of the finger, if necessary continuing through to the opposite side (through-and-through incision).

Abscesses about the fingernails are called *paronychias*. Most are of bacterial etiology and respond to conservative management including antibiotics and drainage. The latter can often be accomplished without anesthesia by separating the adjacent skin from the nail with a scalpel blade or large (18-gauge) hypodermic needle (figure 3-4). Warm soaks are prescribed for a few days to encourage drainage. Sometimes the nail acts as a foreign body, in which case its proximal end must be removed to permit a cure. This is done under sterile conditions and digital block anesthesia. Incise the abscess itself parallel to the long axis of the finger to establish drainage. Pry the proximal end of the nail free with a small hemostat introduced laterally, and use scissors to cut away its proximal third. A small drain may be placed for one or two days if needed to keep the drainage site open. Wound culture and coverage with an antistaphylococcal antibiotic may be indicated in this specific situation, although with most kinds of abscesses antibiotics are usually of no value once the lesion has been opened properly.

Localized herpes simplex infections about the fingertips, sometimes

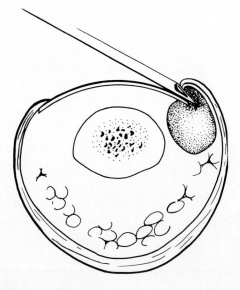

FIGURE 3-4
Drainage of paronychia.

called *herpetic whitlows,* are recognized by their typical appearance: Clusters of small blisters which may break down and become secondarily infected. Tzanck smears or viral cultures can be done if the diagnosis is in doubt. These lesions should be managed conservatively; incision and drainage are not indicated.

Abscesses about the anus are discussed in chapter 14, "Anus and Rectum."

SUGGESTED READING

Davies DM: Benign skin tumours and conditions. *Brit Med J* 290:1128, 1985.

Hill GJ (ed): *Outpatient Surgery,* 2d ed. Philadelphia, Saunders, 1980.

Llera JL, Levy RC: Treatment of cutaneous abscess: A double-blind clinical study. *Ann Emerg Med* 14:15, 1985.

Wolcott MW (ed): *Ambulatory Surgery and the Basics of Emergency Surgical Care,* 5th ed. Philadelphia, Lippincott, 1981.

chapter 4

Skin Trauma

Consultant: ANDREW T. FILAK, JR., M.D.

Most of the minor injuries that patients bring to the family doctor's office or other primary care facility can be handled there with no difficulty if adequate equipment and supplies are on hand. Patients appreciate it when they don't have to be sent elsewhere for care, and the manual exercise of sewing up a laceration can be a welcome change of pace after treating "medical" problems all day.

An appropriate history is important: How did the injury occur? What is the likely extent of contamination? Could there be an unrecognized foreign body in the wound? Might there be an occult fracture or intracranial injury? Does the patient have any preexisting conditions or take any medicine that could complicate the care? What is the patient's tetanus immunization status?

Physical examination should be guided but not limited by the history. When you find one injury, look for another. Check any vital structures—eyes, tendons, nerves, etc.—that may have been damaged. For injuries on the legs of older patients, check arterial pulses and capillary filling time, since impaired local nutrition can greatly delay healing.

LACERATIONS

The management and prognosis of lacerations varies with their location, degree of contamination, and mechanism of injury. Those on highly vascular sites, primarily the head, heal quickly and with little risk of infection. Those on the extremities, especially the legs of patients with compromised arterial circulation, heal more slowly and with a higher complication rate. Wounds contaminated with pathogens or foreign substances are at high risk for infection. Cleanly incised wounds heal more readily than those caused by blunt objects or shearing forces.

Wound Preparation

The skin around a laceration should be washed vigorously with gauze sponges soaked in a diluted germicide-detergent solution (most commonly an iodophor or chlorhexidine). If contamination is severe, do the cleaning in two stages: Wash off the visible dirt, then put on fresh gloves, open a fresh preparation kit, and finish the job. The wound itself should be irrigated with nothing more irritating than normal saline solution. A few dabs with a saline-moistened sponge may suffice in a minor cut with no significant contamination, but careful removal of foreign material and devitalized tissue from contaminated wounds is essential to minimize the risk of infection. Extensive irrigation and mechanical debridement may be needed if, for example, the patient fell on a gravel or blacktop roadway. A large hypodermic syringe and needle, used as a "squirt gun," is often helpful in this endeavor. You may wish to inject a local anesthetic under the raw surface after the initial cleansing but before vigorous decontamination is started. Try, however, to remove the foreign substances with minimal trauma to the exposed tissues.

Crushed or torn tissue heals poorly and is susceptible to infection, so it should be excised under local anesthesia if there is no reason not to do so. Trim away devitalized subcutaneous tissue if there is no risk of taking a nerve, tendon, or artery out with it. Excise crushed skin edges, taking perhaps a 2-mm strip of normal tissue to be sure that fresh, untraumatized edges will be approximated. Partial wound excision may also be indicated if the edges are not perpendicular to the skin surface (figure 4-1). Debridement of facial wounds should be conservative because there often isn't much skin to spare, especially around the eyes, ears, nose, and mouth. Since there is so little redundant skin on the fingers and toes, it's almost always best not to excise any tissue from them that may be viable.

Wound Closure

Once the injured area has been cleaned, made anesthetic, and (if indicated) debrided, drape the area and close the wound. If muscle has been exposed, close the fascia on its surface with absorbable sutures. Correct any gaps in the subcutaneous tissues (dead space) in the same way. If the skin edges cannot be approximated without undue tension, undermine the skin edges or, in extreme situations, prepare skin flaps as described below.

If the skin defect is irregular, its closure may require some ingenuity and trial-and-error suture placement. Place sutures at obvious landmarks first, and then fill in the gaps. Remove and replace any stitches that prove to be misplaced, too loose, or too tight. Dress the injury as described in chapter 2.

Selected small lacerations may be closed with sterile adhesive strips (Steri-strips, butterfly closures, etc.). They can be applied quickly and without anesthesia. They are most suitable for situations in which the wound edges fit together easily and where there is not likely to be much

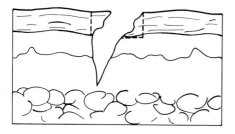

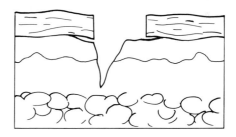

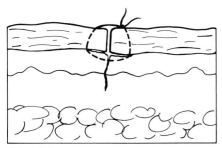

FIGURE 4-1
Correction of wound obliquity.

motion. They are sometimes helpful on irregular finger injuries where placing sutures could increase tissue damage. Fingers so treated should be splinted for a few days.

Lacerations in Specific Locations

The face and scalp have rich blood supply, and lacerations in these areas often bleed profusely. It isn't uncommon to wash away a big blood clot in a patient's hair only to find that the injury that caused it is too small to need suturing. For larger scalp lacerations, especially in children, use absorbable sutures that will fall out by themselves in a few days, making removal unnecessary. Dressings can often be omitted; a spray dressing such as Aeroplast can be used if desired.

Lacerations of the face deserve meticulous repair because the resulting scar will be very visible and, if unsightly, a source of embarrassment to the patient. Remove the sutures after three or four days to minimize the risk of residual "stitch marks." Protect the wound with adhesive strips for a few days afterward. Dressings should not be used around the mouth because they trap food and saliva. Their use is discretionary elsewhere on the face. Since facial skin is often oily, the use of an adherent liquid or spray (Mastisol, compound tincture of benzoin) may be desirable to improve tape adhesion.

Lacerations of the eyelids should be referred unless you are familiar with the specialized techniques needed for their repair. Patients with lid lacerations must be examined carefully for blunt or penetrating trauma to the globe.

Lacerations of the ears have a high risk for infection if the cartilage is exposed. If you elect to repair one, irrigate it well, trim the cartilage conservatively, and close the wound with small, superficial stitches. Devise a dressing that supports the ear gently and follows its anatomic contours, both laterally and medially. Avoid excessive pressure on the dressing. Major ear lacerations should be referred.

Lacerations of the edges of the lips require special care to be sure that the vermilion border is approximated accurately with no step-off. Marking landmarks with an indelible pen may make a precise repair easier.

With through-and-through lacerations of the lips and cheeks, close the mucosal laceration first with absorbable sutures (unless it is minor and falls into position well). Irrigate the wound well from the outside, and then close the skin defect. If a mucosal laceration was caused by the patient's own teeth, it should be repaired carefully to minimize the resulting scarring; a scar which rests against the edges of the patient's teeth may remain tender for a long time.

Minor tongue lacerations are often left alone; they heal well and the cosmetic result is relatively unimportant. Larger lacerations which could leave a cleft in the tongue when they heal should be closed with absorbable sutures.

Finger lacerations require special attention to insure optimum functional recovery. Check carefully for evidence of nerve, tendon, or arterial injury. Some digital nerve injuries are too small to justify repair, but with the advent of microsurgical techniques it has become possible to repair many of them. If an anesthetic area will be left after skin healing, instruct the patient that the area will lack sensation for weeks to months and therefore will be abnormally susceptible to injury. The management of tendon lacerations is beyond the scope of this book; if you find one in a setting where a properly trained surgeon is not available, close the skin, tell the patient that he has a major injury that requires special attention, and make an appropriate referral.

Profuse bleeding from extremity wounds can be controlled temporarily by a tourniquet until more definitive hemostasis is possible. The easiest way to do this is with a blood pressure cuff. Inflate it to a pressure just above the patient's systolic blood pressure, and maintain it at that level for a few minutes until the source of bleeding is identified and controlled.

You can use a rubber band or a piece of Penrose tubing as a finger tourniquet, but one very important precaution must be observed: If a rubber band that has been wrapped around a finger for hemostasis should be forgotten and left on under the dressing, necrosis and sloughing of the finger can occur. The only safe way to use a rubber band as a tourniquet is to wrap it around the finger doubled and hold it in place with a hemostat. The instrument is too large to be incorporated in the dressing and forgotten.

As a general rule, finger lacerations should be treated conservatively with a minimum of debridement, few if any buried sutures, and only enough skin stitches to hold the tissues in place until healing occurs. Sterile adhesive strips can often be used advantageously on irregular finger lacerations if good hemostasis can be achieved. The tapes will not stick to bloody skin, however.

Lacerations across the nailbed have been managed in many ways. Some advocate keeping the fingernail in place as a splint. Try not to place sutures in the nailbed if good approximation of the wound can be achieved otherwise. If the distal phalanx was fractured as part of the injury and the distal bone fragments are palpable in the wound, it's often wise to excise them to diminish the risk of infection.

Tips of fingers are often sliced off, leaving a raw surface devoid of epithelium. The repair is accomplished under digital block anesthesia, using a tourniquet as described above if necessary. Any bone protruding into the wound is trimmed back with a rongeur. If the amputated skin is

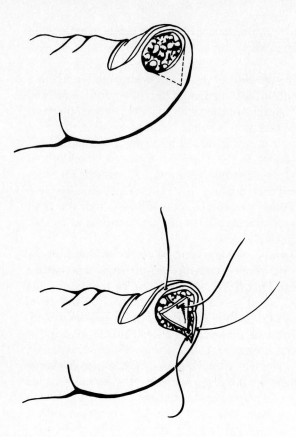

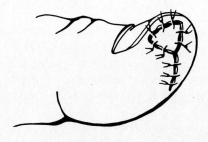

FIGURE 4-2
V-Y repair of fingertip.

available, it can be used as a free graft; clean it off in sterile normal saline solution, trim all the fat off its underside, and sew it loosely in place. In some cases it may be desirable to cut a small full-thickness skin graft from the volar aspect of the forearm and sew it in place.

Another method of repair is the V-Y technique (figure 4-2) in which a triangular area of the pad of the finger is mobilized and advanced to cover the fingertip wound, after which the skin is closed in a Y pattern.

A key to success in the management of finger injuries is immobilization, usually with an aluminum splint incorporated in the dressing. The less the finger moves, the less risk of infection and delayed healing. Immobilization must not be carried on too long because of the risk of permanent reduction in joint mobility. One week of fixation is usually sufficient, and it should rarely be prolonged beyond two weeks.

Avulsion-lacerations of the pretibial area are often sustained by children falling against a step or other fixed object, often with a shearing force that tears the skin rather than cutting it (figure 4-3). There is often gross contamination with gravel, grass, and/or dirt. They are prone to infection but with meticulous attention to detail most of them will heal primarily. The key steps include thorough debridement and irrigation of the wound, excision of the skin margins if this can be done without creating undue tension, applying a compression dressing and inserting a drain for twenty-four to forty-eight hours to minimize serum accumulation, and immobilizing the knee joint with a plaster splint for a few days.

CONTAMINATED WOUNDS

All wounds sustained outside a surgical suite are contaminated to some extent. The important variables are the part of the body injured, the extent of the contamination, the interval between injury and treatment, and the extent to which the tissues have been devitalized. To overstate

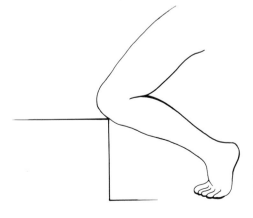

FIGURE 4-3
Mechanism of pretibial laceration.

the obvious, a clean incised wound of the face sustained two hours ago on a sharp knife has a better prognosis than the previously described avulsion laceration of the leg, expecially if six or eight hours elapse between trauma and repair. The old benchmark of six hours as the dividing line between a laceration that can be closed primarily and one that must be managed by the open method is reasonable, with more time allowed on head cuts, less on those with devitalized tissue, and none at all on some grossly contaminated ones.

If you feel obliged to close a wound of marginal risk for infection, pay particular attention to the previous comments about irrigation, immobilization, and other principles of wound care. Avoid buried sutures; close subcutaneous space with vertical mattress sutures if necessary. Use as few stitches as possible, and don't pull them tight. Use sterile tape strips rather than sutures if possible. Inspect the wound frequently, and instruct the patient to return at the first sign of fever or local pain.

In the face of gross contamination or other high-risk situation, use the open method of treatment with delayed suturing. Clean and debride the wound. Place a layer of fine-mesh gauze in the base of the wound, fill the space with fluffed gauze, and create a bulky dressing. Leave it undisturbed for three to five days unless there is evidence of gross infection. If the wound looks good at the time the dressing comes off, suture it. If not, debride any nonviable tissue and repeat the process until it either becomes suitable for stitching or closes secondarily.

Human bites should never be sutured because they are heavily contaminated with multiple pathogens, many of them anaerobes. An innocent-looking puncture wound of the hand caused by striking an opponent about the mouth may progress to an acute necrotizing soft-tissue infection, with devastating consequences. Obtain cultures from these injuries, and then treat them with irrigation, debridement, immobilization in the position of function with a bulky dressing, elevation, and generous doses of antibiotics (e.g., cloxacillin 500 mg qid). In this setting the antibiotics are not considered prophylactic and should be continued for at least a week. If a joint or tendon is involved, consider hospital admission for intravenous antibiotics and surgical consultation.

Human bites of the face also require irrigation, debridement, and antibiotic coverage. Some feel that delayed suturing (after four days) or early loose closure with monofilament sutures may be permissible. Buried sutures should not be used unless the wound has been completely excised.

People who have sustained human bites may deny the cause in an attempt to avoid personal embarrassment or possible legal complications. Thus the physician must consider the possibility whenever the location and circumstances are suspicious.

The bites of domestic animals are somewhat less likely than human bites to become infected, so the rules given above can be applied somewhat less strictly. Selected bites which have been well irrigated and which are free of devitalized tissue can be sutured if they are *in areas other than the hand.*

SKIN GRAFTS

Small split-thickness grafts can be cut with a razor blade and used to cover relatively small skin defects caused by deep burns or other trauma. The most common donor sites are the anteromedial aspect of the thigh and the volar aspect of the forearm. The appropriate depth is best learned under supervision. Removal of the graft should cause punctate bleeding but subcutaneous fat should not appear. Full-thickness grafts are occasionally used for fingertip injuries; they are discussed above in the section "Lacerations in Specific Locations."

Flaps are occasionally used to fill skin defects; one doesn't often need to use them in office surgery, but it's wise to know a few of the techniques. A rotated flap is prepared as shown in figure 4-4. Plan its size carefully to fill the defect with only slight tension, and mark the planned incision with an indelible pen. Incise the skin along the line you have prepared, and cut it free from the underlying tissue. Suture the flap into its new bed, and close the area from which it was rotated as shown. Advancement flaps are prepared in a similar way, but with a different topological arrangement (figure 4-5).

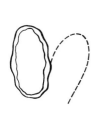
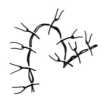

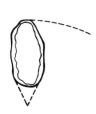
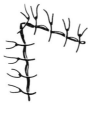

FIGURE 4-4
Rotational flaps.

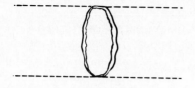

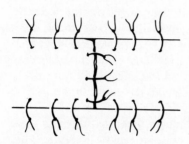

FIGURE 4-5
Advancement flap.

PUNCTURE WOUNDS

The most common type of skin puncture wound is a foot injury caused by stepping on a nail; these will be discussed at some length. Punctures associated with animal bites have been discussed in the section "Contaminated Wounds." Other types of puncture wounds associated with foreign bodies are discussed in the following section. Needle stick injuries are a major cause for concern among nurses and laboratory technicians but will not be discussed here because the care of the wound itself is a minor issue compared to management issues arising from the possibility that the needle stick may spread infection.

Recent publications on the subject of puncture wounds tend to favor aggressive management including excision of the wound, vigorous irrigation, frequent soaks, and the use of oral antibiotics. The author has found no controlled studies on the value of these methods and no consideration of the possibility that aggressive management may actually increase the risk of morbidity. For example, repeated soaking of an injured foot may defeat the normal protective effect of a scab, and inappropriate antibiotic therapy may encourage the overgrowth of antibiotic-resistant pathogens. In the absence of good data we must fall back on an analysis of the relevant facts:

1. The typical puncture of the foot is caused by stepping on a nail while wearing a shoe. Nails used in house construction are typically 2 to 4 mm in diameter, and the effective size of a puncture wound is typically smaller because of the normal elasticity of the skin. The depth of penetration is usually unknown because the nail is removed

before arrival at the medical facility, but it could be a centimeter or more in adults, depending on whether it enters directly or obliquely and whether it passes between bones or strikes one of them. Thus one is confronted with a wound which has a functional diameter of no more than a millimeter or two, with a depth that may be many times that amount. Forceful irrigation of such wounds seems as likely to spread contamination along fascial planes and possibly tendon sheaths as to remove it.

2. Foreign matter can be picked up by the nail as it passes through the shoe and the stocking. There can also be a wiping action in which debris on the nail may be cleaned off by the shoe, stocking, and skin. Thus the amount of contamination carried into the wound is unknown. In one study retained foreign matter was found in 26 of 887 pediatric patients (2.9 percent) with foot puncture wounds. The largest number of these were fragments of socks and rubber-soled shoes.

3. Cellulitis occurring soon after a puncture wound is usually caused by staphylococci. *Pseudomonas aeruginosa* causes most cases of late osteomyelitis. There is little evidence that the incidence of the former is reduced by prescribing antibiotics. The latter is a ubiquitous organism which causes infection primarily in compromised tissue and which responds only to a few antibiotics which must be given parenterally.

4. It has been the author's experience that almost all patients who present with cellulitis have been soaking the foot at home, and in many cases family members have been probing the wound.

5. Excising wound margins sounds like a good idea, but the skin of the foot is thick and there is little of it to spare, so there is a risk of closing such an incision under excessive tension. One would like to see some controlled studies to support the often-expressed opinion that the excision of ordinary puncture wounds reduces morbidity.

Based on the foregoing considerations, a review of established practice, and personal experience with the conservative management of puncture wounds, the author recommends the following approach to puncture wounds of the foot.

1. Obtain a complete history: Did the injury occur in a clean environment or in a muddy barnyard? What was the patient wearing on the injured foot? How many hours have elapsed since the injury? Does the patient have any other health problems that could affect the risk of complications, such as peripheral arterial insufficiency or poorly controlled diabetes, or any condition or treatment compromising the immune system? What is the patient's tetanus immunization status?

2. Clean the skin about the injury well with an antiseptic-detergent preparation, one time only.

3. Inspect the wound for evidence of contamination, and clean out any that is visible.

4. The decision to excise the wound should be individualized. Excision is more likely to help the patient if significant tissue destruction is visible and if the history indicates that probing and irrigation are indicated. A 4-mm dermal biopsy punch may be used to excise the puncture wound while disturbing the surrounding tissues as little as possible. Let it close spontaneously.

5. Explore the wound with a blunt probe, and irrigate it with a syringe only if the history suggests a reasonably high risk of foreign body contamination. Try to avoid traumatizing the tissues or spreading contamination by overenthusiastic treatment. Use only sterile saline solution for irrigation, avoiding iodine-containing preparations and other cytotoxins.

6. Apply an elastic bandage without much compression, both to encourage immobility and to discourage ill-advised tampering with the wound by patient or family. Leave the dressing undisturbed for about three days.

7. Have the patient use crutches for a similar period to further encourage immobility of the foot while the body's normal defenses cope with any microscopic contamination that may have occurred.

8. Antibiotics are indicated only for high-risk situations. Prescribe them according to sound principles for wound prophylaxis, as opposed to treatment for established infections: Start as soon after the injury as possible, maintain generous blood levels, and stop them in two or at most three days.

9. In selected high-risk situations, especially where bone, cartilage, or a joint has been injured, consider prophylactic administration of parenteral antibiotics effective against *Pseudomonas*.

10. Order tetanus immunization as indicated.

SUBCUTANEOUS FOREIGN BODIES

In questioning a patient who may have a subcutaneous foreign body, determine the nature of the object, the circumstances under which the injury occurred, and the time interval from injury to examination. Try to estimate the velocity with which it entered and its trajectory in relation to the skin surface. Inquire about preexisting health problems that may influence the outcome, and check on the patient's tetanus immunization status.

The wound of entrance is frequently quite small and innocent-appearing. In some circumstances the foreign object may be palpable under the skin, but often one can only guess at its location. Metallic foreign bodies are easily detected by x-ray. Automobile glass and some other types of glass are radiopaque, but wood is usually radiolucent unless covered by paint. Xeroradiography may bring out some otherwise invisible objects. CT scanning will demonstrate wood and may be worth the expense on occasion. Placing one or more markers on the skin will help with the localization process. A small lead marker is often taped over the entrance wound. Bent paper clips can be affixed over the area as additional guideposts. Sometimes sterile hypodermic needles of different lengths are inserted into the tissues as markers.

Consider the nature of the foreign body in planning treatment. Metal and glass objects are well tolerated by the tissues; they may occasionally be left in place if they are not near vital structures and if locating them for excision is likely to be difficult. They may also be left if there are too many of them to make removal practical (shotgun pellets, for example). Wood, on the other hand, is more irritating and should almost always be removed. This may be easy if the wood is sound and can be lifted out in one piece, but it may be arduous if it is rotten. Sea urchin spines are quite irritating if left in place and should be excised. Injuries caused by explosions (fireworks, for example) and those in which paint, solvents, or other irritating substances are injected into the tissues under high pressure may have serious consequences and generally should be referred.

The location of the foreign body may also influence management. Those which are near bones, tendons, nerves, and blood vessels require more prompt and definitive management than those at a distance from such structures. Foreign objects near an open fracture may predispose to serious infection. Low-risk foreign bodies can sometimes be removed in an office surgery, but they may be much more difficult to locate than anticipated. When any doubt exists as to whether you can find and remove the object without undue risk to the patient, arrange for definitive care in a surgical suite. The procedure is rarely an emergency; it should be performed methodically in a proper setting.

There are three circumstances under which you may elect to leave a subcutaneous foreign body in place. First, a patient may have other, more serious medical problems which must take priority. Second, there may be significant local infection which should be treated before removal is undertaken. Third, if the object is made of a relatively bland substance (a steel chip, for example) and is embedded deeply but at a distance from vital structures, you may elect not to remove it. This decision should be documented in the medical record and discussed with the patient, of course.

The technique of removal will vary with the location and nature of the object. Start by localizing it as precisely as possible, using x-rays and markers if necessary. Gentle probing of the entry tract may be indicated. Obtain adequate local anesthesia, make the smallest incision that will permit adequate access, and dissect down to the object. If it is palpable through the skin (a sewing needle, for example), you may be able to make just a small nick in the skin, push the object up into the wound, and pull it out with forceps. Irrigate with sterile normal saline before closure if multiple small fragments are present. Place a drain for a day if it was necessary to dissect through much tissue. Close the wound with sutures or sterile tapes unless there is major contamination. Be sure the patient's tetanus immunizations are up to date.

The author has had no experience with the removal of sea urchin spines from the sole of the foot, but has been told that the best way to do this is to take a small dermal punch, cut out the spine and a surrounding small circle of skin *en bloc,* and let the resulting defect close spontaneously. This procedure might also be helpful with other painful foreign bodies embedded in the thick skin of the soles and palms.

SUPERFICIAL SPLINTERS

Patients will occasionally request removal of a wood or metal splinter which has become lodged within or just below the skin. A tiny mass which happens to be embedded in the pad of a finger or in another sensitive location may cause significant worry for the patient even if it is so small that it cannot be seen with the naked eye. You can avoid wasting time pursuing such objects if you have the proper equipment on hand and use it effectively. The first necessity is a good head magnifier, used with adequate bright lighting. The second is a proper splinter forceps which has not been damaged by misuse.

Start by cleaning the area well with soap and water, both to minimize the risk of introducing infection into the wound and to soften the epithelium. No anesthesia will be necessary if the splinter is superficial. If it is deeper and there may be a need to cut the skin to gain access to the foreign body, local infiltration with lidocaine or a similar agent may be in order. If the lesion is near the surface of the skin, you may need to do nothing more than shave the epidermis gently with a scalpel blade to unroof the splinter track and then flick the offending object out. If it is deeper, it may be necessary to trim the skin a bit or cut down vertically to the foreign body to be able to grasp it with the splinter forceps.

If the foreign body is composed of metal or sound wood, there is no need to explore the tract after the object is removed. If it is of rotted wood or other friable material, there may be concern about possible residual fragments. You will have to use clinical judgment in deciding how far to go in exploring for these. In some cases the wisest course is to avoid further disruption of tissue and tell the patient that there is a small chance that a remaining fragment will make itself known in a few days by causing local inflammation. The patient should of course return if this occurs. No dressing or aftercare is needed if the splinter did not penetrate the basal layers of the skin. If the lesion was deeper, apply a dry dressing for a couple of days to protect the area until it closes over.

Similar principles are used in the treatment of a splinter under a fingernail. Start with soap and water. If the object can be grasped with splinter forceps, it probably can be removed without anesthesia. Since local infiltration into the fingernail area is difficult and painful, a digital block is usually preferable. Unroofing a wedge of the nail with scissors or a scalpel will sometimes help you gain access to the end of the splinter. Leaving the fingernail long after the procedure would permit the accumulation of dirt which could predispose to infection, so cut it short.

EMBEDDED FISHHOOKS

Fishhooks are difficult to remove from the skin for the same reason fish find them hard to dislodge from their mouths: The hooks have barbs near their tips that resist backward movement. Many methods have been devised for removing hooks; each may be appropriate at times.

The most commonly used technique is advancing the tip through the skin (under sterile conditions and after injecting a local anesthetic agent), cutting off the tip and barb with a wire cutter, and backing the shank out (figure 4-6). Lacking a tool strong enough to cut the hook, one can accomplish the same objective by squeezing the barb flat against the shank with a sturdy needle holder or pliers.

A second method, with which the author and consultant have had no experience, involves the gentle introduction of a large-bore hypodermic needle into the entrance wound beside the shank, advancing it to form a sheath over the barb, and then withdrawing the fishhook and the needle together (figure 4-7).

A third method is shown in figure 4-8. Place the body part in which the hook is embedded on a firm surface. Loop a piece of sturdy twine around the curve of the hook, and grasp it firmly in your right hand. Hold the shank between the thumb and middle finger, as shown, to disengage the barb from the subcutaneous tissue. Give a strong horizontal jerk on the string with your right hand to pull the hook out.

If none of these methods is successful, it may be necessary to cut down

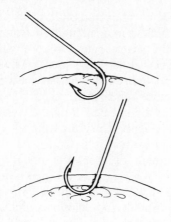

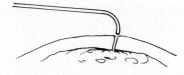

FIGURE 4-6
Fish hook removal, first method.

to the point with a scalpel, extract the hook, and close the resulting incision with a few sutures.

ABRASIONS

Most abrasions of modest extent are best treated by cleaning them up and leaving them exposed to the air until a hard scab forms. The cleaning may be extensive and may have to be done under local anesthesia if foreign material has been ground into the abraded skin. Use a head magnifier, good light, a scalpel, and plenty of normal saline solution. In some situations, particularly where the abraded area must be covered by clothing, a nonstick pad and absorbent dry dressing may be applied.

CONTUSIONS

Bruises characteristically look their worst a few days after injury, when free blood works its way to the surface and its various breakdown

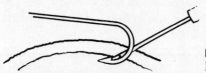

FIGURE 4-7
Fish hook removal, second method.

products show their green and yellow colors. The treatment at this stage is largely reassurance. In rare occasions one must test the patient for a bleeding disorder, although the appropriate tests may be abnormal in healthy patients during the time a contusion or hematoma is resolving. If a contusion or hematoma is recognized shortly after injury, cold applications or compression dressings may be used to minimize their extent.

HEMATOMAS

When a hematoma forms after injury, a decision must be made as to whether to evacuate it or not. Small hematomas will usually resolve by themselves or else become small fixed masses of no significance. Fresh hematomas can sometimes be evacuated with a sterile syringe and large needle, but use meticulous technique to avoid iatrogenic infection. Hematomas that have clotted cannot be drained competely by aspiration, of course, although it is often possible to draw out enough bloody fluid to confirm the diagnosis. Old blood is hygroscopic, and if it is not removed completely, the hematoma is likely to form again after aspiration. The only way to empty a clotted hematoma is by incision and drainage. Try to locate the incision at the lowest part of the mass so that it can drain by gravity.

Hematomas of the external ear must be drained promptly. This lesion is discussed in the section "Ear Problems" in chapter 7.

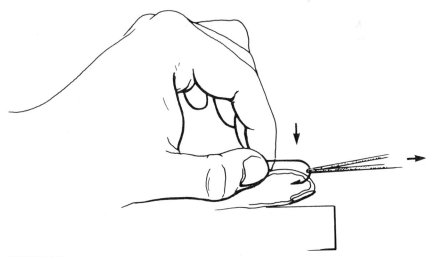

FIGURE 4-8
Fish hook removal, third method.

BLISTERS

Most blisters should be left intact. The longer the interval from onset to rupture, the more mature will be the epidermis on its base. Some writers speak of blister fluid as an ideal culture medium, but the author has never seen infection in an intact blister. If a blister is so large as to interfere with the patient's activities, one may try nicking and deflating it under sterile precautions.

BURNS

Some burns can be managed very well in a primary care setting. Others, which may have an unfavorable prognosis and/or require more skilled care, should be referred out. The choice depends on many factors:

1. **The Appearance of the Burn.** Classically, burns have been described as first degree (epidermal damage only), second degree (damage, short of total destruction, to the epidermis and dermis), and third degree (full-thickness destruction of the skin). It is more practical to think clinically of first degree (erythema only), superficial second degree (blistering and/or desquamation over a viable, pink dermis), and deep (dead tissue present, whether demonstrably full-thickness or not). First-degree burns, however painful initially, will heal without scarring or disability if they are not converted to deeper types by mismanagement or secondary injury. Superficial second-degree burns will heal if they do not become infected. Deep burns carry a worse prognosis and require more specialized care.

2. **The Size of the Burn.** As a rough rule of thumb, burns involving no more than 10 to 15 percent of the body surface (less for small children and the elderly) may be managed in an ambulatory setting, while larger ones should be treated in a hospital. Estimation of the area of smaller burns is facilitated by remembering that the palm of one hand has an area of 1.25 percent of the total for that patient, at any age. The *rule of nines* is a useful tool for estimating the extent of larger burns in adults (figure 4-9). Proportions are different in children; in infants the head constitutes 20 percent of the total surface.

3. **The Location of the Burn.** Burns of the hands tend to lead to disability from contractures and decreased joint mobility; this can also be a consideration in major burns about other joints. Burns of the perineum are difficult to keep clean. Facial burns may involve the eyes or, if due to steam or hot gases, damage to the lining of the

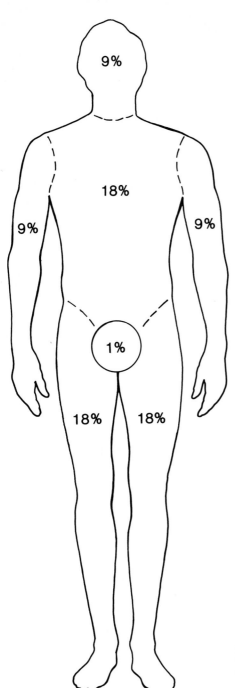

FIGURE 4-9
The rule of nines. Note that the back accounts for another 18 percent.

respiratory tract. All patients with suspected respiratory tract burns require hospital care.

4. **The Cause of the Burn.** Chemical burns and high-voltage electrical burns are often much more severe than they seem at first. Chemical burns should be treated immediately with prolonged irrigation with water to wash out every possible trace of the offending agent. With electrical burns it is essential to look for a second burn elsewhere on the body. For example, a patient who touched an exposed high-voltage wire may have an obvious burn on the hand, and also a less evident one on the leg or foot where the circuit was completed to the ground. Electrically burned patients are at risk for renal damage from myoglobinuria and should receive appropriate prophylactic care in a hospital.

5. **The Age and Health of the Patient.** Small children and the elderly tolerate burns less well than other patients. The prognosis is worse in those chronically ill or poorly nourished. Preexisting infection in the patient or a personal contact may predispose to infection in the burn.

6. **Associated Injuries.** Examine the patient for other injuries such as fractures or damage to internal organs if the burn was sustained in an industrial, motor vehicle, or other accident.

7. **Personal and Family Resources.** The safety and feasibility of ambulatory burn care are influenced by the the alertness and reliability of the patient and family and by the quality of their relationship with the treating physician.

Ambulatory Treatment

Immediate cooling of the burned tissue will reduce thermal damage and may prevent a minor burn from becoming a major one. Depending on the site, this can be accomplished by applying cold, wet towels, by immersing the part in cold water, or by whatever other means is readily available. The sooner it is started, the better. If it has not been done before you see the patient, apply cold for a few minutes as soon as the patient arrives.

Once the pertinent history has been obtained and it is certain that no contraindications exist, consider giving an injection of an analgesic agent if the patient is in severe pain. Do not inject local anesthetic agents into burned tissues. If it is apparent from the initial examination that the patient should be treated in a hospital, cover the burned area with a sheet and arrange for transportation immediately. Definitive care should be left to those who will be responsible for the patient henceforth, except that intravenous fluids should be started before transportation if there is evidence of shock or if a long trip will be necessary. Associated problems such as fractures or airway problems should of course be managed appropriately. The remainder of this discussion applies only to patients judged appropriate for ambulatory management.

Gentle cleansing of the skin with bland soap and water is in order, but do not cause the patient more pain than necessary or further damage burned tissue by overenthusiastic scrubbing or by using agents containing alcohol or other irritants. Broken blisters and other debris should be debrided conservatively. Intact blisters should be left alone in all but unusual circumstances.

First-degree burns may be dressed for comfort, especially in areas that may rub against clothing. Apply a layer of fine-mesh antistick gauze, followed by bulk in the form of fluffed gauze squares and an appropriate top dressing. However, most of these injuries can be left open; a bland ointment may be applied as the patient desires, although maceration of the skin must be avoided. Ordinary vegetable shortening (Crisco, other brands), applied sparingly, works well. Anesthetic burn creams carry a risk of allergic sensitization. Antibacterial preparations are not indicated.

Superficial second-degree burns, in which viable, pink dermis is seen, may be treated by sterile occlusive dressings changed every two to four days. It is impossible to prevent bacterial colonization in their surface, but if further insult to tissues and invasion by pathogens can be prevented, most will heal without incident within two weeks. Cleansing and application of dressings are done under sterile conditions. A fine-mesh antistick dressing material such as Adaptic is applied to the skin, and then sterile gauze is applied in the form of squares, fluffs, large pads, and/or bulky roll materials such as Kerlix. Stockinette or a compression bandage may be applied loosely if the burned area is relatively small, but it is essential to allow for edema to accumulate in the burned area without compromising the circulation through excessive pressure. A sling or other means of elevating the injured part should be used when appropriate. Neither topical nor systemic antibiotics are indicated, except in unusual circumstances.

Burns in which deeper tissue has been devitalized take longer to heal, are more likely to become infected, carry a less favorable prognosis, and require more intensive and skillful treatment. Scarring may lead to restriction of joint motion or, if circumferential, to circulatory embarrassment. Thus the decision to treat a deep burn in the primary care office should be made only after weighing all aspects of the case. It can be undertaken if no more than 3 to 5 percent of body surface is involved, if patient and family are prepared to provide the necessary home treatment, if no other contraindications exist, and if the physician is in a position to follow the patient closely. Initial treatment is the same as for superficial second-degree burns: Gentle cleansing, conservative debridement, and a bulky sterile dressing. In two or three days, after the initial inflammatory reaction has started to subside, a program of home treatment begins. Twice each day the burned area is washed gently, perhaps in a shower, and any loose debris is removed. Any involved joints are run through a full range of motion to retain mobility. The area is then gently dried. An antimicrobial ointment such as mafenide or silver sulfadiazine is applied generously to the burn with a gloved hand or tongue depressor. Depending on the burn's location, it may either be left open or covered with a simple dry dressing.

The injury is examined by the physician every few days and the rate of healing carefully noted. Local debridement of separating burn eschar may be indicated on occasion. If any area of full thickness skin loss too large for spontaneous closure (more than about 2 cm in least diameter) is identified, arrangements should be made for skin grafting.

Once the skin is closed, the twice-daily treatments are discontinued and long-term rehabilitation begins. The new skin is kept soft with bland ointments and protected from bright sun and other irritants. Physiotherapy may be prescribed to correct any restrictions of joint motion (it may be indicated earlier in some burned patients). In some cases elective orthopedic surgery will be needed to overcome contractures. Wearing elastic bandages or stockings for as long as a year may help to keep scar formation to a minimum.

The risk of tetanus is high for all but trivial burns, and appropriate immunization is necessary.

SUGGESTED READING

Arons MS, Fernando L, Polayes IM: *Pasteurella multocida*—the major cause of hand infections following domestic animal bites. *J Hand Surg* 7:47, 1982.

Callaham M: Prophylactic antibiotics in common dog bite wounds: A controlled study. *Ann Emerg Med* 9:410, 1980.

Dagher FJ (ed): *Cutaneous Wounds*. Mount Kisco, N.Y., Futura, 1985.

Edlich RF, Rodeheaver GT: Puncture wounds. *Compr Ther* 10(6):41, 1984.

Fitzgerald RH, Cowan JDE: Puncture wounds of the foot. *Orthoped Clin N Amer* 6(4):965, 1975.

Moylan JA: Outpatient treatment of burns. *Postgrad Med* 73(3):235, 1983.

Pories WJ, Thomas FT: *Office Surgery for Family Physicians*. Boston, Butterworth, 1985.

Smoot EC, Robson MC: Acute management of foreign body injuries of the hand. *Ann Emerg Med* 12:434, 1983.

Tobin GR: Closure of contaminated wounds: Biologic and technical considerations. *Surg Clin N Amer* 64(4):639, 1984.

chapter 5

Dermatological Procedures

Consultant: RICHARD S. MORAITES, M.D.

POTASSIUM HYDROXIDE PREPARATIONS

The presence of fungi in skin lesions can often be demonstrated by scraping off a bit of the superficial epithelium, mixing it with potassium hydroxide solution (KOH) to dissolve normal skin elements, and looking for hyphae and spores under the microscope. The tool used for scraping should not be too sharp; the edge of a second glass slide or the back of a scalpel blade will do. If you want to examine the specimen immediately after it is obtained, it may be necessary to heat the preparation on the slide to dissolve the keratin, especially if 10% KOH is used. Heating is usually not required with a 30% solution or if the preparation is allowed to stand for an hour or two. The organisms are most likely to be found on the advancing edge of tinea lesions and on the underside of nails involved with onychomycosis. Use of the microscope is discussed in chapter 17, "Laboratory Procedures."

WOOD'S LIGHT

Various fungi which cause dermatoses (sometimes *Microsporum* spp, occasionally *Malassezia furfur*) may fluoresce when exposed to ultraviolet light. It's useful to keep a small ultraviolet lamp designed for this purpose (Wood's light) at hand as an aid to the diagnosis of these conditions. Its use is simple: Darken the room, shine the light on the lesions, and examine for spots of fluorescence on the affected hairs. Look carefully; lint and other foreign objects may also fluoresce.

A Wood's light can be used for other purposes, including diagnosis of certain uncommon pigmentary disorders, pseudomonas infections in burns, and (with fluorescein instillation) corneal abrasions. The urine of patients with porphyria cutanea tarda also may fluoresce.

DIAGNOSTIC PROCEDURES FOR SCABIES

Sarcoptes scabei is a tiny arthropod (about 0.25 mm in length) that causes intense itching as it burrows into the superficial epithelium. A presumptive diagnosis of its presence can be made by the history and finding groups of papules (often with excoriation) in typical sites such as finger webs, wrist and elbow creases, waist, and the inguinal and perineal areas.

This presumption is strengthened by demonstrating the characteristic burrows made by the mite in the superficial epidermis. Use a head magnifier (loupe) and good light. Apply mineral oil to suspected lesions, especially over the elbows and other dry areas; this will tend to make the burrows, and sometimes the mites within, more visible. An alternative and more dramatic technique is to apply ordinary fountain pen ink to suspect areas, wash it off with an alcohol swab, and look for ink-stained burrows. They can be very short or an inch (25 mm) or more in length.

A more definitive diagnosis may occasionally be needed. This requires microscopic demonstration of the eggs, egg casings, scybala, or adult mite. Apply mineral oil to suspected lesions on the hands, wrists, or elbows to identify those most suitable for examination. Look for fresh, uninflamed burrows which have not been scratched. The most productive technique for obtaining a specimen for examination is to squeeze the skin containing a burrow gently between your thumb and index finger and shave the superficial epithelium off with a scalpel. Anesthesia is not required, but the patient may experience some discomfort. Do not cut deeply enough to cause bleeding. Put the specimen on a glass slide, cover it with mineral oil, apply a cover slip, and examine it under the microscope's lowest magnification. A less reliable but technically easier approach is to apply mineral oil to the lesion, scrape it with a scalpel blade, and examine the scrapings as described above.

Scabies may present quite a different clinical picture in debilitated and immunocompromised patients: a nonpruritic scaling rash that contains large numbers of mites which can be spread easily to health care workers (this is called Norwegian scabies).

TZANCK SMEAR

The blisters of herpes simplex and varicella-zoster infections frequently contain multinucleated giant cells which can be demonstrated under the microscope. This method is not as reliable or specific as viral culture, but the cost is lower and the results can be obtained quickly.

Use a head magnifier and wear gloves. Select an intact blister, and wash the area with an alcohol swab. After it dries, unroof the lesion with fine scissors or a scalpel. Blot away the blister fluid (this is the time to obtain a culture if that is indicated). Scrape the base of the lesion gently with a scalpel, and spread the harvested material on a glass slide. Apply Giemsa's, Wright's, or toluidine blue stain (see chapter 17, "Laboratory Procedures"). Examine the slide with the oil immersion lens, looking for multinucleated giant cells. The same procedure can be used, although with a lower yield, with pustular lesions. Tease the scab away with the scalpel blade, and obtain the specimen from the bed as described above.

Viral and fungus cultures may be useful for specific diagnosis, but the availability of appropriate laboratory services varies from one community to another. Consult your pathologist.

WARTS

Warts are collections of abnormal hyperplastic epithelium caused by local infections with the papovavirus. The clinical course is long because an effective immune response to the agent does not occur. Warts are not dangerous but may bother the patient in a number of ways: In certain locations (fingers, genitalia) they may become irritated and tender. On the sole of the foot ("plantar" warts) their presence causes accumulation of keratin and a "stone-in-the-shoe" sensation. Their unsightly appearance disturbs some patients. Since the lesions are benign and usually resolve in a year or two, it is important not to use overly aggressive treatments. This is particularly true on the foot, where a temporarily uncomfortable condition could be replaced by a permanently tender scar. The available options for treatment include the following:

1. **Application of Keratolytic Agents.** These do not cure the wart because they do not destroy the layers of the skin where the virus lives, but they remove hyperplastic keratin and may make the patient more comfortable as the problem runs its course. Effective agents include keratolytics dissolved in collodion (Duofilm, etc.) and "corn plasters" containing salicylic acid. The latter are available in preshaped pads or in large sheets which can be cut to the desired size and shape. The patient applies the agent until the keratin softens and then rubs it off.

2. **Excision of Keratin.** One can shave the excessive keratin from a plantar wart or, with a bit of practice, learn to remove it *en bloc*. Start at the edge of the mass, and define a plane of lessened tissue density at its junction of the normal skin. Lift up on the keratin, and gently dissect it away from the underlying tissue. This technique is also effective with corns. Patients with steady hands and good vision can sometimes shave their own corns and plantar warts, but this

should not be encouraged, especially in older patients with diminished vision and impaired circulation, because of the risks associated with cutting too deep.

3. **Application of Podophyllin.** Podophyllin, most often supplied in 20% concentration in compound tincture of benzoin, is often effective with perineal warts and those about the fingers. It is irritating and may be washed off by the patient after a few hours. Efforts should be made to keep it off adjacent normal skin. Repeat treatments are sometimes needed.

4. **Destructive Treatments.** Warts can be destroyed by cryotherapy and fulguration; these modalities are discussed later in this chapter. Those on the surface can be removed with a dermal curette, after which their bases are treated with light cryotherapy or fulguration. Sharp-knife excision is usually not indicated because of the resulting scarring; treatment of warts generally should not leave a scar.

5. **Suggestion.** Various methods of magical removal of warts have been recommended, and there are reliable people who assert that they work. One approach is to state dogmatically, in the presence of the patient and family, that the wart will be gone by a certain holiday which is some months in the future.

6. **No Treatment.** Many patients will be best served by no treatment other than explanation of the nature of the condition.

MOLLUSCUM CONTAGIOSUM

Like warts, the lesions of molluscum contagiosum are caused by local infection with a virus. They present as somewhat translucent umbilicated papules in locations suggesting direct person-to-person transmission, most often in children. They can be removed by curetting and fulguration or other locally destructive treatments. They are relatively resistant to cryotherapy.

CRYOSURGERY AND FULGURATION

Carefully controlled destruction of superficial tissue is often useful in patients with benign epidermal lesions. It can also be used, by those with special training and equipment, for certain malignancies. *Fulguration* (destroying tissue with a high-frequency electric current) can be performed with inexpensive spark generators which require little maintenance. *Cryosurgery* (local tissue destruction by freezing) is a better method in practices with sufficient volume to justify purchasing the more expensive equipment and supplies needed. Local anesthesia, usually by injection, is required for fulguration (exception: tiny lesions that can be treated in a second or less). Cryosurgery can usually be performed without anesthesia, which is especially advantageous with small children. With either technique the necrotic tissue usually separates and sloughs off in a few days with little local reaction and, if the procedure was performed properly, little risk of infection or other complications.

Both techniques are contraindicated when the nature of the lesion being treated is unknown. In some cases (warts, for example) the diagnosis causes little difficulty, but in others a tissue biopsy is needed before treatment. Use special caution in areas where cosmetic results are important, such as around the mouth and nose and on exposed skin of deeply pigmented patients. Rare absolute contraindications to cryosurgery include cryoglobulinemia and Raynaud's disease.

Cryosurgery

Dermatologists perform cryosurgery chiefly with liquid nitrogen, purchased every few days from commercial suppliers and kept in specially insulated containers. For most lesions small amounts of the liquid are applied with loosely wound cotton applicator sticks. The use of liquid nitrogen is impractical in smaller primary care practices; the material is inexpensive, but it evaporates and it would be used too seldom to justify the time required to purchase it and keep it constantly in stock.

Practices which provide gynecological care are often equipped with gun-type cryosurgery units which use nitrous oxide or other compressed gas for the treatment of chronic cervicitis. These units can also be used for skin lesions. They are relatively expensive, and the cost of the gas cylinders is significant, but storage of the equipment and gas between uses presents no problem. These devices usually come with tips of varying sizes and shapes; if possible, treat each lesion with a tip that covers the lesion and very little of the surrounding normal tissue. Use standard water-base surgical lubricant (KY, other brands) to ensure good thermal contact between the instrument and the tissue.

Ethyl chloride spray and disposable cans of freezing sprays can be used to provide cold anesthesia, but they do not create a low enough temperature to be effective for cryosurgery. Caution: Ethyl chloride is highly flammable.

The benign lesions most frequently treated with cryosurgery by primary physicians include warts, seborrheic keratoses, and actinic keratoses. Leukoplakia and mucoceles of the lip also respond well. The freezing application time varies from five to twenty seconds, with a maximum "thaw time" (total time from the start of freezing until the ice ball melts) of about thirty seconds. Molluscum contagiosum doesn't respond as well; these lesions are better treated by spraying them for a few seconds to produce anesthesia and then removing them with a dermal curette.

The treatment of warts varies according to location and other characteristics. Since they are epidermal lesions, it is neither necessary nor desirable to destroy deeper dermal tissues in their treatment. Raised warts (as, for example, on fingers) can be treated in a straightforward manner by freezing them as described above. With plantar warts it's often helpful to remove as much of the overlying keratin as possible, either by careful paring with a scalpel or by repeated application of a keratolytic agent, such as salicylic acid plasters, before freezing them. Mosaic warts respond poorly to cryotherapy, as they do to other forms of therapy. Periungual warts are difficult to manage with cryosurgery, or, for that matter, with any other form of treatment. One can try paring off overlying keratin and freezing the wart for about five seconds.

It may take as few as two or as many as six treatments to destroy a wart. For best results the interval between treatments should be no more than three weeks.

Lesions on the ears, nose, and eyelids respond well to cryosurgery, usually with excellent cosmetic results, but one needs experience and judgment to determine the appropriate duration of treatment. It is always better to err on the side of undertreatment rather than take a chance on damaging underlying tissues; you can always retreat if necessary.

The skin responds to cryosurgery as it would to any other thermal injury. Aching is perceived both during the initial cooling process and during the thaw. Erythema and edema appear after the treatment, and there is often blistering. Pain medication is seldom required, but patients should be told what to expect. Brief follow-up visits should be scheduled to monitor the healing process and to determine the need for retreatment.

Fulguration

Simple damped-wave electric spark generators (Hyfrecator, other brands) are inexpensive and require little attention between uses. They can be used to destroy warts, although their use on plantar warts is usually not recommended because overenthusiastic treatment can lead to a permanently tender scar. Fulguration is suitable for certain other benign lesions such as molluscum contagiosum. Seborrheic keratoses may also be treated if care is used to control the depth of treatment. Sterility is not required because the spark kills any microorganisms in its path, but the skin should be mechanically clean. Local anesthesia, usually by injection, is normally required. There is generally little or no tissue reaction; the cauterized tissue becomes hard and gradually sloughs off.

To fulgurate a typical raised wart, first inject the area with a local anesthetic agent such as lidocaine. Since the spark causes heat, and the patient may perceive heat as painful even if pain neurons are blocked, good anesthesia is required. For best results make an initial subcutaneous injection, and once that has started to work, make a second intradermal injection for more profound anesthesia. If the wart is relatively small, it may be destroyed systematically by a small, well-controlled spark. If it is larger, remove most of the wart with scissors or a dermal curette and then electrocauterize its base. Apply aluminum chloride or ferric subsulfate (Monsel's) solution as needed for hemostasis. If the patient reports pain at any stage, slow down the rate of treatment to minimize heating of tissues. In most cases the lesion should not be dressed after treatment since a hard, dry eschar provides excellent protection during the subsequent epithelialization process. Advise the patient that the area may be washed normally but that it should be dried promptly afterward.

Certain hazards must be kept in mind when using fulguration. The spark can ignite organic liquids such as alcohol or ethyl chloride. Also, treating undiagnosed lesions with electrocautery is as hazardous as treating them with cryosurgery.

REMOVING TICKS

Ticks attach themselves to humans and pets by their mouths and then secrete a cement which increases the strength of their attachment. Since they carry a variety of diseases, it is important to remove them promptly but in a way that does not risk causing infection in either the person bitten or the one who does the removing. Squeezing the tick's body can increase the risk to both parties.

Using a small forceps, grasp the tick as close to the mouth parts as possible, and gently but firmly pull it loose without twisting or jerking motions. If it is necessary to remove ticks in a field situation distant from medical equipment, hold a sheet of plastic material between your fingers and the tick, grasp it as close to the mouth parts as possible, and make every effort to avoid squeezing its body. Wash your hands and the bite site with soap and water. Do not touch the tick or permit others to do so.

INTRALESIONAL INJECTIONS

Acne cysts, localized psoriasis lesions, and certain other skin problems can be treated with intralesional injections of insoluble, slowly absorbed corticosteroid drugs. Keloids can also be treated during the early months of their development, but with greater difficulty and less assurance of good results. The preparation most often used is triamcinolone acetonide suspension, 10 mg/ml, diluted 1:1 or 1:2 with normal saline or lidocaine solution, depending on whether a temporary local anesthetic effect would be useful. It is injected with a tuberculin syringe and a fine (25- to 27-gauge) needle. The volume may vary from 0.05 to 0.25 ml per lesion, depending on size; larger volumes may be needed with keloids. Multiple lesions may be injected at one sitting, but the total dose should not exceed 20 mg. Repeated injections at one- to two-week intervals may be needed. Patients must be selected and doses planned with care because large and/or repeated injections of the drug may cause systemic corticosteroid effects. The material is injected into the dermal layers of the skin; the skin should rise slightly at the time of the injection. Subcutaneous injection would greatly increase the risk of unsightly tissue atrophy.

SUGGESTED READING

Amundson LH, Caplan RM: The skin and subcutaneous tissues, in Taylor RB (ed): *Family Medicine: Principles and Practice,* 2d ed. New York, Springer-Verlag, 1983, pp. 1074–1144.

Estes SA: Diagnosis and management of scabies. *Med Clin N Amer* 66(4):955, 1982

Knight PJ, Reiner CB: Superficial lumps in children: What, when and why? *Pediatrics* 72:147, 1983.

McBurney EI: Diagnostic dermatologic methods. *Ped Clin N Amer* 30(3):419, 1983.

Needham GR: Evaluation of five popular methods for tick removal. *Pediatrics* 75:997, 1985.

Romm FJ: Treatment and outcome of warts. *J Fam Pract* 22:373, 1986.

Sober AJ: Diagnosis and management of skin cancer. *Cancer* 51:2448, 1983.

Solomon AR, Rasmussen JE, Varani J, et al: The Tzanck smear in the diagnosis of cutaneous herpes simplex. *J Amer Med Assoc* 251:633, 1984.

Zacarian SA: *Cryosurgery for Skin Cancer and Cutaneous Disorders.* St. Louis, Mosby, 1985.

chapter 6

Eye Procedures

Consultant: DAVID N. TUCKER, M.D.

Ocular procedures must be approached with care because therapeutic misadventures or missed diagnoses can lead to catastrophic blindness. One should not hesitate to refer a patient whose diagnosis is uncertain or who is not responding promptly to treatment. However, properly trained family physicians can and should perform a number of ophthalmic procedures as part of their daily practices. The keys to success in such techniques are good lighting, good magnification, and steady hands. The last of these is often aided by letting the heel of your hand rest on the patient's forehead or cheek as your fingers work.

EQUIPMENT AND SUPPLIES

The direct ophthalmoscope is a hand-held device for eye examination which contains a series of lenses and a light source. The lenses, of gradually increasing positive and negative diopter strength, are mounted in a circle on a small disc which can be turned to rotate one lens at a time over a small viewing aperture. The light, whose intensity is controlled by a rheostat, is directed by a prism system so that its axis is almost parallel to your visual axis as you look through the aperture and lens. Many ophthalmoscopes have a system for changing the character of the light beam. By rotating a small collar, you can select any of the following types of light:

1. Unrestricted incandescent light, suitable for most purposes.
2. Small spot of light, useful where you wish to reduce the total amount of light striking the retina.
3. Slit light, to improve identification of certain ocular lesions, such as the presence of cells in the anterior chamber of the eye in patients with iritis.
4. Red-free (green) light, to increase the visibility of microaneurysms and other vascular abnormalities of the retina.
5. Grid, to permit semiquantitative measurement of retinal lesions.

If an ophthalmoscope becomes difficult to use after it has been in service for a time, any of the following problems may be present: The light bulb may have developed black deposits which reduce its light output; replace the bulb. The prism may have been jarred out of proper alignment, causing the beam of light to be misdirected; have the instrument repaired. The lenses may have gotten dirty; have them cleaned, or do it yourself if you have enough time, talent, and patience.

The best approach to vision testing, if your practice volume justifies the space and the investment, is the use of a Keystone, Titmus, or other vision testing machine. These instruments offer distant, near, color, fusion, depth perception, and phoria testing in a single efficient package. The traditional wall-mounted eye chart, with progressively smaller letters corresponding to different levels of visual acuity at a distance of 6 meters (20 feet), provides a satisfactory measure of distant vision.

Charts for the testing of illiterate patients, consisting of lines of a broadened letter "E" in different sizes and turned in different directions, are also available. These charts should be viewed at a measured distance of 20 feet and must be well illuminated if results are to be accurate. Samples of small type in various formats can be obtained for testing of near vision. Books containing Ishihara color test plates are available to test color vision.

A standard-focused floor- or ceiling-mounted examining lamp provides adequate illumination for eye examinations. You should have a method of reducing the overall light level in an examining room for opthalmoscopic work and fluorescein testing of corneal lesions.

You will need either a small pen-size flashlight or a standard otoscope light to test pupillary reflexes and to check for shallow anterior chambers.

Good magnification is essential when you examine eyes for injuries or foreign bodies. This is best accomplished by head-mounted binocular magnifiers. The most common type fit snugly around your head and have their lenses positioned so that you can use them without removing your eyeglasses. Another type is designed to be clipped to eyeglass frames.

A sharp sterile spud is used to remove corneal foreign bodies and to scrape away rust rings. The handiest tool for this purpose is an ordinary disposable 3-ml hypodermic syringe with a relatively large (18- or 20-gauge) needle.

Small sterilized swabs are used to remove foreign bodies found at the inner canthus or under the eyelids. Standard commercial applicator swabs are much too large. Make your own by twisting small wisps of cotton-ball material around toothpicks.

A special pen-size flashlight with a dark blue filter can be used to bring out the fluorescence of fluorescein-stained corneal lesions.

A Schiotz tonometer may be used to screen for glaucoma. These instruments come in a fitted case with add-on weights, spherical test surface, and instructions. Ordinary pipe cleaners work well for cleaning the inside of a tonometer. Acetone and cotton balls should be available for decontaminating the foot and plunger tip before and after each use.

A pinhole device, perhaps nothing more than a sheet of opaque plastic with a tiny hole in its center, is useful for identifying refractive errors in children and for differentiating refractive from retinal problems in older patients. They can be purchased commercially or be home-made.

Fluorescein solutions should not be used for eye examination because pseudomonas organisms grow in them readily. The most practical source of fluorescein is prepackaged filter paper strips impregnated with the agent (Fluor-i-strips, etc.).

Sterile solutions for instillation in the eye are available either in plastic squeeze bottles or in small single-use containers. The former are more economical; the latter carry a lower risk of contamination, especially in practices where it is difficult to be sure that the highest standards of aseptic technique are followed at all times. The following additional drugs and supplies should be stocked:

> Topical anesthetic solution such as tetracaine 0.5% (Pontocaine, other brands)
> Short-acting mydriatic agent such as tropicamide (Mydriacyl) or 2.5% phenylephrine (Neo-synephrine)
> Squeeze bottles of eye-irrigating fluid

Some physicians stock additional drugs such as antibiotics, steroids, or miotics in ointment or drop form, but in most cases their risks exceed their benefits.

> Individually packaged sterile eye patches
> Metal eye shields
> Applicator sticks (to evert eyelids)

VISION TESTING

Some aspects of vision should be tested routinely; others can be pursued more selectively. Although less sophisticated approaches will suffice in some circumstances, a vision testing machine, as described in the previous section, will prove to be a good investment in most practices. One or more staff members will have to be trained in its use and monitored from time to time to ensure that the reported test results are uniformly reliable. The following parameters are normally tested:

Distant visual acuity is most often tested by measuring the patient's ability to read letters of standard size, either through the optical system of a testing machine or on a wall chart. The patient is simply instructed to read from the largest letters toward the smaller ones until no longer able to discriminate letters. The standard reporting system is based on what a "normal" person can read at a distance of 20 feet: A subject who tests 20/30 is able to read at 20 feet what one would be expected to read at 30 feet. Each eye is tested individually. This is accomplished mechanically in testing machines. When using a wall chart, one hands the patient something to hold over one eye while the other is being checked. Opaque plastic occluders are available, or one can use anything suitable which happens to be at hand, such as a scratch pad. Be sure the patient does not press on the eyeball during the occluding process, since this would interfere with subsequent testing of that eye. Testing both eyes together may aid in the recognition of diplopia; because of their double vision such patients characteristically see less well with both eyes together than with the better eye alone. Patients who wear glasses or contact lenses should be tested wearing them and again after they have been removed.

Testing of *near vision* is less well standardized. Vision testing machines measure one's ability to read type of progressively smaller size at a predetermined distance. With other protocols the size of the type is constant, and you move it back and forth to see at what distances the patient can read it.

In *phoria testing* each eye is presented with a different visual image, so arranged that they should be perceived by the brain as being in a certain relationship to one another. If the eye muscles are not well balanced, the two eyes will become oriented in somewhat different axes and the patient should describe an image to the tester that is different from the standard. A simple approximation of this test may be achieved by the "cover test" which is done as follows: The patient sits facing you, and you ask him or her to gaze at your nose or at something on the wall behind you. Hold an occluder or your hand close to the patient's face for a few seconds in a way that blocks vision with one eye. Then remove the obstruction, watching the previously occluded eye carefully. Repeat the procedure on the other side. If there is significant *heterophoria* (tendency for unequal extraocular motion), the affected eye will tend to drift off axis while it is occluded and jump back to correct orientation when your hand is removed. This testing is important for preschool children and for any patient who reports diplopia.

Color vision testing with pseudoisochromatic plates is a sensitive measure of genetic color blindness, a sex-linked characteristic found almost exclusively in male subjects. However, the degree of penetrance varies widely, and you will often have to decide on clinical grounds whether a patient is too impaired to fulfill a certain role. For example, one might be unable to discriminate subtle color differences well enough to work with multicolored telephone communications cables but still be able to identify red, yellow, and green traffic lights reliably. Keep some colored objects at hand which you can use to quiz patients about their ability to detect reasonably bright colors.

Eye testing of high quality can and should be done on children prior to school entry. Many children will have been taught to recognize letters; the rest can be tested with "E" charts or special pediatric charts with familiar shapes (ball, house, etc.). If a child tests poorly, have him or her repeat the test looking at the target through a pinhole. Visual acuity of subjects with refractive errors improves when the effective aperture is small, in the same way that a camera's depth of focus becomes greater when the iris is stopped down to f/22.

THE OPHTHALMOSCOPE: OPTICAL CONSIDERATIONS

The physics of visual focusing is reviewed here briefly because it contributes to an understanding of ophthalmoscopy and visual function. The numbers are oversimplified for illustrative purposes.

The focusing ability of a lens is measured in diopters; the number of diopters represents the reciprocal of the focal length in meters. For example, a 2-diopter lens has a focal length of 0.5 m, or about 20 inches. Diopter numbers of lenses are additive; for example, if you put a 2-diopter lens and a 3-diopter lens together, the effect is that of a 5-diopter lens (focal length 40/5 = 8 inches). This applies to negative (concave) lenses as well: Combining +3 and −2 lenses creates a +1 effect.

The normal human eye has a depth of about 1 inch, so the normal ocular lens must have a focal length of about 1/40 meters, or a power of 40 diopters if it is to focus on objects at a distance. The human lens is flexible; its shape changes and its optical power increases when it needs to focus on nearby objects. However, this flexibility diminishes with age at a predictable rate, so older people need eyeglasses to see nearby objects even if their distant vision remains normal; this constriction of focusing range is called *presbyopia.*

If an individual's eye is of normal depth but the lens measures 41 diopters, the eye will not focus at infinity and distant objects will appear blurred. However, the eye will focus at a distance of 1 meter and the patient will see nearby objects well. This condition, which may be of widely varying severity, is called *myopia,* or nearsightedness. It is corrected by eyeglasses with negative (concave) lenses (figure 6-1).

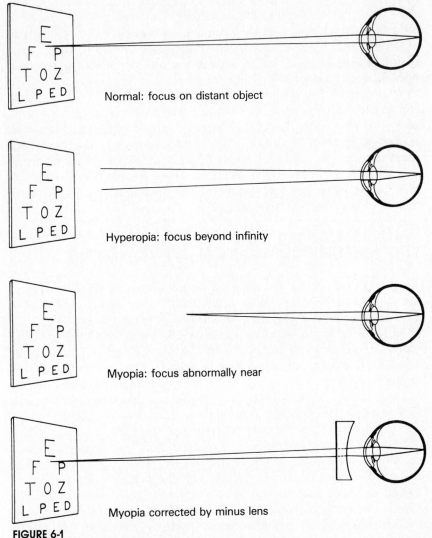

Normal: focus on distant object

Hyperopia: focus beyond infinity

Myopia: focus abnormally near

Myopia corrected by minus lens

FIGURE 6-1
Refraction and retractive errors.

If one has a 39-diopter eye lens, the eye will focus beyond infinity, and the intraocular muscles will need to bend the lens to bring objects into focus. This condition is called *hyperopia* or farsightedness; it is corrected by positive (convex) lenses.

There is always a zone of sharp vision in front of and beyond the theoretical point of focus. The depth of this area can be quite shallow when the pupil is dilated and the effective lens aperture is great. It becomes progressively greater as the pupil constricts and can be made quite deep by looking through a pinhole. Thus the fact that objects may appear sharper in bright than in dim light has a physiological basis: The iris closes down in bright light, increasing the depth of focus. Some people with uncorrected refractive errors habitually try to increase their depth of focus by squinting, which reduces the effective aperture.

The optical system of the opthalmoscopic examination includes (in order) the patient's retina, the patient's lens, the opthalmoscope lens, the examiner's lens, and the examiner's retina (figure 6-2). If both people have normal refractive systems, there will be good visualization with the ophthalmoscope's optical system set at zero diopter. If either or both persons have a refractive error, an appropriate corrective lens can be dialed into position in the instrument.

These considerations lead to a practical hint: If you have difficulty getting the retina in focus because of a refractive error in the patient, ask to borrow the glasses for a moment. Look through the ophthalmoscope and the patient's lens at a distant object, and rotate the dial on the instrument until the object comes in focus. Read the dial, reverse the sign, and you have a close approximation of the patient's refractive error. For example, if it takes a +4 lens to see the distant object through the patient's glasses, you conclude (assuming that your own refractive error is negligible) that the patient needs a −4 correction. Dial that number on the opthalmoscope, and you should be able to see the patient's retina.

The discussion to this point has assumed the absence of a significant degree of *astigmatism,* or nonspherical refractive abnormality. If you suspect that the patient's glasses may be corrected for this condition, hold them at arm's length and rotate them as you look through them. If you see a "barrel" type of distortion that rotates as the glasses are turned, you know that the glasses have a correction for astigmatism. If the condition is severe, you may not be able to see the retina well at any setting.

USING THE OPHTHALMOSCOPE

Start by explaining the procedure to the patient. Since it is difficult for most people without biological science training to visualize the anatomy of the eye, you may wish to use a simple drawing. One useful analogy is to compare the eye to a Ping-Pong ball with a small hole in one side. The examination requires you to look through this hole and the lens that

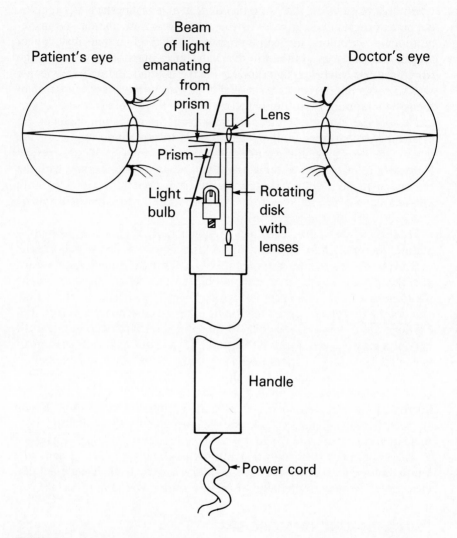

FIGURE 6-2
Optics of the ophthalmoscope.

covers it to visualize some structures on the inside of the back surface of the ball. You can point out that this is the only place in the body where you can look directly at blood vessels without invasive surgery and that the appearance of these structures may reflect the condition of vessels elsewhere in the body.

Proper examination of the fundi requires dilatation of the pupils. This can be done safely if a few precautions are taken to identify the small number who should not receive mydriatic drops. If the patient has had an intraocular lens implant, be sure that it is not of a type that can be dislodged by dilating the iris. The risk of precipitating narrow-angle glaucoma has often been used as an excuse for not dilating pupils, but it can be prevented by two simple steps. First, inquire about any history of painful attacks of decreased vision that might have represented subacute narrow-angle glaucoma. Second, check for shallow anterior chambers by shining a penlight tangentially over the iris from the temporal side. If the iris protrudes anteriorly, it will cast a shadow medially, the so-called volcano sign (figure 6-3). The use of mydriatics is contraindicated in patients with head trauma or certain other neurological conditions because of the importance of being able to watch pupil size, but that is rarely

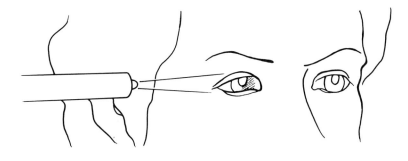

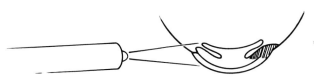

FIGURE 6-3
Volcano sign of protruding iris.

a problem in office practice, or indeed in the care of most hospital patients.

Use a short-acting mydriatic such as tropicamide. If you apply two drops in each eye at the start of a general physical examination, the pupils will usually have dilated by the end of the exam and you can finish up with funduscopy. Pull the lower lid down by downward traction with your thumb, have the patient look upward, and drop the medicine in the conjunctival sac (figure 6-4). Both patient and physician usually remove their eyeglasses before ophthalmoscopy, but this is not mandatory. You may want to leave your glasses on if you have difficulty reading the numbers on the instrument without them. If the patient is astigmatic, you may get a better look at the retina if he or she leaves the glasses on. Contact lenses need not be removed.

Have the patient seated, usually on an examining table, with eyes at about the same level as yours. Ask the person to fix his or her vision on an object on the wall behind you: the corner of a picture, a light switch, or, if necessary, an "X" you have created with plastic tape. Tell the patient to continue looking in that direction even if your head gets in the way.

Dim the room lights; one way to do this is to turn on your examining lamp, aim it at a light-colored wall, and turn off the overhead light. Turn the ophthalmoscope lamp on, but not to full brightness; use the lowest level of light that will let you see the retina well. Set the lens system at +15.

To examine the patient's right eye, hold the ophthalmoscope in your right hand and look through it using your right eye. Start a foot or so from the face, check to see that the light is aimed properly, and move in until the eyelids and cornea come into focus. If the patient's upper eyelid appears to be getting in the way, place your opposite hand on his or her forehead and elevate the upper lid with your thumb. Turn the lens disc a step at a time to bring each structure you encounter into focus in its turn: cornea, iris, lens, and finally the retina. Follow the arterial tree to the optic disc, noting its color, the sharpness of its margins, and the size and character of cupping. Check to see if it is in focus with the same lens as the adjacent retina or if it requires a different magnification (indicating depression or elevation). Follow each major arteriole outward, noting abnormalities such as narrowing, tortuosity, arteriovenous nicking, emboli, and any hemorrhages or exudates. Finally, examine the macular area. If you have trouble locating it, ask the patient to look directly at the light. This is the area most sensitive to light, and if you have not used a mydriatic, you may be unable to visualize the macula because of reflex constriction of the iris sphincter. Repeat the procedure with the other eye.

An eye examination should be done in the first month or two of life as

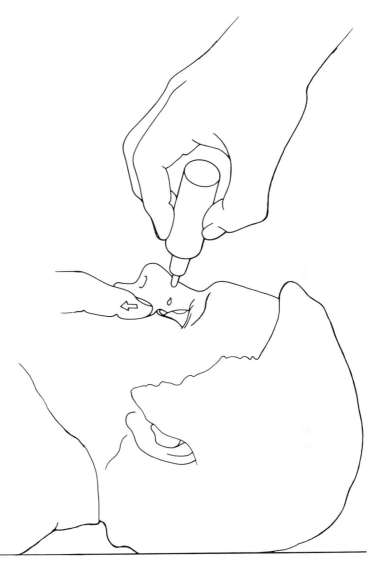

FIGURE 6-4
Instilling eye drops.

a part of well baby care. Examine each newborn with a small light held near your own eyes to demonstrate the "red reflex" of light reflected from the infant's retina. Note the small spot of light reflecting from the cornea; it should be in the same relative position in both eyes if the child does not have an extraocular muscle problem. The iris should be visible, the pupils equal in size. Most infants will lie still for an ophthalmoscopic examination in the first few months of life. Some newborns will have retinal hemorrhages near the disc; these should resolve promptly in a few weeks.

TONOMETRY

Indications for use of the Schiotz tonometer, a hand-held device for estimating the intraocular pressure, have been the subject of controversy. On one hand, chronic glaucoma is a significant but insidious cause of preventable blindness. On the other hand, there is some normal day-to-day variation in intraocular pressure, the Schiotz instrument is less accurate than the applanation tonometers used by ophthalmologists, and only a minority of patients with relatively high intraocular pressure will prove to have glaucoma. Many patients over 40 years of age, the group chiefly at risk for glaucoma, have already undergone tonometry by an opthalmologist or prevention-oriented optometrist. Tonometry in the primary physician's office may be indicated for patients over 40 years of age in whom the test has not been done elsewhere, especially if there is a family history of open angle glaucoma. Contraindications to the procedure include recent ocular trauma, infection, and sensitivity to local anesthetic agents.

The Schiotz tonometer is a small but precisely made device consisting of a hollow stem with a footpiece whose contour matches that of the eyeball; a weighted plunger which is free to move up and down within the stem; a lever system which indicates the level of the end of the plunger in relation to the footplate; a collar used to hold the instrument which is free to slide up and down the stem; and some additional small weights that can be put on the upper end of the plunger (figure 6-5). The tonometer can be disassembled for cleaning.

Explanation to the patient should stress that it is important not to move the eyes while the procedure is being done and that you will numb the eyes so that there is no discomfort. Some apprehensive subjects will find it difficult to keep their eyes open when the instrument is being moved into position, so you will want to move slowly and be as reassuring as possible.

The patient lies supine on an examining table. A drop or two of an anesthetic solution such as tetracaine 0.5% is applied in each eye. If there is not a suitable visual "target" on the room's ceiling for the patient to look at, have the patient hold one arm out straight upward, make a fist with the thumb protruding, and use the thumbnail as an object on which to fix the eyes. You can move the arm slightly so that the pupils are looking directly upward.

Assemble the tonometer, and check its accuracy by resting it on the test

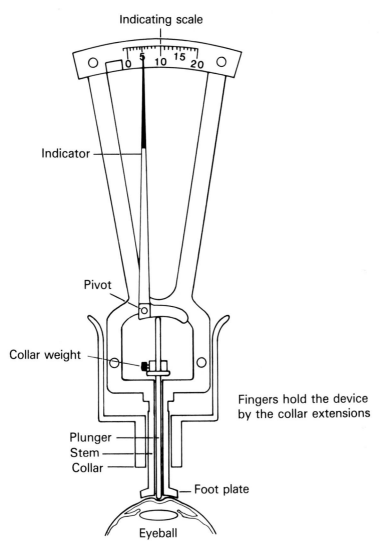

Indicating scale

0 5 10 15 20

Indicator

Pivot

Collar weight

Fingers hold the device
by the collar extensions

Plunger
Stem
Collar

Foot plate

Eyeball

FIGURE 6-5
Schotz tonometer.

sphere built into the case; the indicator should show zero. Wash the footplate and plunger with a cotton ball that has been wetted with acetone; let it dry thoroughly before proceeding with the examination. If practical, stand at the head of the table so that you can let the heel of your hand rest on the patient's forehead during the procedure. Hold the instrument by the collar, hold the lids of one eye open with the thumb and index finger of the opposite hand, and set the tonometer gently down on the eye. The collar should not touch the top or bottom of the stem, so that the weight of the instrument rests on the eye. Note the scale reading; if it is higher than 6, add a weight to the plunger so that the reading is in the desired range. Repeat the procedure on the other eye (figure 6-6).

Clean the stem and footplate before putting the instrument away. Disassemble it periodically for more thorough cleaning.

Use the conversion table with the instrument to determine the intraocular pressure corresponding to the scale reading and weight used for the test.

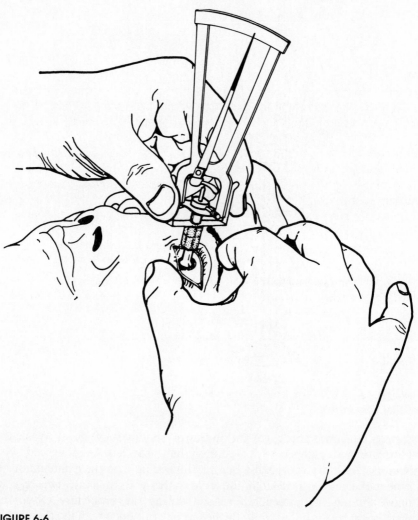

FIGURE 6-6
Method of using tonometer.

Readings above 20 mmHg or significant difference in pressure between the two eyes is considered an indication for ophthalmological referral.

OCULAR TRAUMA

For the purposes of this discussion it is assumed that the patient is examined supine on a standard examining table, which is the usual procedure in primary care. The use of slit lamps and examining chairs, which requires a larger capital investment than family doctors need to make, is not discussed here.

The initial examination of the traumatized eye may be very deceptive, especially if an adequate history is not obtained. Penetrating foreign bodies may leave almost invisible wounds. Retinal detachments may go undetected unless you suspect their presence and look for them. Make every effort to determine the nature of any forces that were applied to the area, the nature and velocity of any incoming foreign bodies, and the patient's previous visual acuity. Eyelid lacerations are difficult to repair in a way that will give a good end result; most should be referred to an ophthalmologist or plastic surgeon.

If initial inspection suggests that the injury may be so extensive that the services of an ophthalmologist are required (examples would include penetrating wounds, blowout fractures of the orbit, and major lacerations), do nothing more to the eye except to apply a protective dressing. Be careful not to put any pressure on the globe, and incorporate an eye shield in the dressing if there is any possibility of a penetrating injury. Alkali burns represent an exception; see discussion at the end of this chapter in "Chemical Burns of the Eye."

Physical Examination

With patients suitable for care by the primary physician, the visual acuity, at least distant vision, should be checked before any other treatment is started. This information should be carefully recorded since it may have both medical and legal significance.

A local anesthetic agent may be instilled to relieve pain and *blepharospasm* (spasmodic closure of the eyelids) before starting the examination. Use a good light, but direct it to the eye from an angle to minimize the patient's discomfort. Wear a head magnifier. Separate the lids gently and inspect the eye methodically. The lower lid is easiest to evert, using simple downward traction with your thumb just below the lid margin. The upper lid is larger and more difficult to evert because of the fibrous tarsal plate which must be turned before the area can be adequately visualized.

Grasp the upper eyelashes between the thumb and index finger of one hand, and hold an applicator stick against the outside of the upper eyelid with the other. Ask the patient to look down. Then lift upward on the eyelashes while you apply gentle downward pressure with the applicator to "flip" the tarsal plate and turn the lid upward. With practice you can learn to evert an eyelid using only the fingers of one hand: Grasp the eyelashes with your thumb and index finger and lift, while applying downward pressure on the tarsal plate with your middle finger. Once the upper lid is everted, you can hold the lashes against the supraorbital ridge with your thumb while you use the other hand to complete your examination. When the procedure is completed, ask the patient to look up; doing so will usually turn the tarsal plate back into its normal position.

Ocular Foreign Bodies

Free ocular foreign bodies are most often found under the upper lid near its margin. They are usually removed easily with a small cotton swab made with a toothpick. Anesthesia is usually indicated but may be omitted if removal is easy. If you are unable to find a foreign body in a patient who feels that one is present, there are two possibilities:

1. The object may be so small or so translucent that you can't see it; sometimes it's helpful to wipe the area of the eyelid (not the cornea) where an object is most likely to be found.
2. Often, however, a foreign body sensation persists after the object has been washed away by tears or normal lid motion. Anesthetize the eye and patch it overnight, and the symptoms are usually gone the next morning.

Many free ocular foreign bodies, especially multiple small objects, can be removed by irrigation after instillation of an anesthetic agent. Turn the patient's head part way to the side, place a kidney basin to catch the irrigating solution, retract the lids as previously described, and wash the object(s) away with a gentle stream of isotonic irrigating fluid from a plastic squeeze bottle.

Foreign bodies on the cornea are usually adherent but can be picked off with a sharp instrument. The most practical choice for this purpose is an ordinary 3-ml hypodermic syringe with a 20-gauge needle attached. Instruct the patient to fix his or her gaze upward, having the person use the thumb of one hand as a "target" if necessary. Sit at the head of the table, and let the heel of your hand rest on the patient's forehead for stability. Work slowly and carefully under good light and magnification. If the foreign body contains iron, there will often be a rust ring around the site where it was lodged; scrape it away with the needle tip. Remove as much of the rust as you reasonably can, but it is better to leave a trace of rust than to take the risk of puncturing the cornea.

The eye should be patched if a corneal foreign body was removed or if the cornea has been scratched by the motion of a foreign body under the upper lid. If you elect to use a topical antibiotic, apply it in the conjunctival sac as previously described. Use two standard eye patches to achieve adequate thickness of the dressing. Fold the inner one in half for a better fit and firmer pressure. Tape them firmly in place so that the lids will not try to open under the dressing; this is best accomplished by securing one end of the tape to the patient's cheek, pulling obliquely upward, and securing the other end to the middle of the patient's forehead (figure 6-7). Patching is not necessary after removal of a free foreign body which caused only minimal irritation of the conjunctiva.

Caution the patient with a patched eye that depth perception and side vision will be impaired, either of which may interfere with the ability to drive a motor vehicle or to negotiate stairs safely. Tell the patient that the patch may be removed on arising the next day if the eye is comfortable at that time. Always schedule a follow-up visit the day after removing an ocular foreign body or treating a corneal abrasion. Most of the time the cornea will repair itself overnight, but there is a small risk of infection, erosions or ulcers, or residual foreign material.

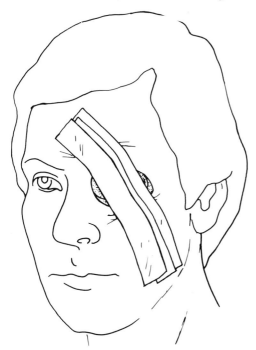

FIGURE 6-7
Method of patching the eye.

Removal of an ocular foreign body provides an ideal "teachable moment" for the discussion of eye safety. Your discussion should motivate the patient to use eye protection faithfully in the future to prevent a recurrence of the pain and risk to eyesight which foreign bodies entail.

Corneal Abrasions

Corneal abrasions occur in varied settings: A small child may innocently stick a finger in someone's eye during play; a branch may whip into a patient's face during a walk in the woods, and of course many foreign bodies cause abrasions as described in the previous section. Blepharo-spasm is usually present and often severe. It may be necessary to evert the lower eyelid and instill a drop of local anesthetic solution before adequate examination can be performed.

Once the eye is numb and the lids have relaxed, the examination can proceed. Inspect the lids, lid recesses, and globe for foreign bodies and evidence of trauma. All but the most severe corneal abrasions are invisible to the naked eye. In order to see them, you will need to instill fluorescein, a fluorescent dye which stains traumatized tissue but not the intact conjunctiva. This material, which is supplied on small, sterile-wrapped paper strips, should be applied only after the eye has been anesthetized. For convenience you can apply a drop of local anesthetic solution to the end of the paper strip and then touch the moistened paper to the conjunctival strip. Ask the patient to close the eye and look in all directions to distribute the material over its surface. Let the patient know that the material will impart an orange tint to his or her vision for a few minutes. Then dim the room lights and view the cornea and remaining conjunctiva with a small ultraviolet light, looking for the typical green fluorescence wherever the surface of the eye has been denuded. The treatment of corneal abrasions is simply to protect them with an eye patch until they heal, which may happen in as little as eight hours depending on their size.

Chemical Burns of the Eye

The initial treatment of chemical burns of the eye is irrigation, irrigation, and irrigation. A topical anesthetic may be instilled. Start with a plastic squeeze bottle of irrigating fluid, flushing out the recesses under the upper and lower eyelids. Hang up a bottle of an isotonic intravenous fluid, and let it run through the IV tubing to continue the irrigation. Hold the lids open manually or with a lid retractor if necessary. These patients should always be managed by an ophthalmologist after the initial treatment.

SUGGESTED READING

Ervin-Mulvey LD, Nelson LB, Freeley DA: Pediatric eye trauma. *Ped Clin N Amer* 30(6):1167, 1983.

Newell SW: Management of corneal foreign bodies. *Amer Fam Phys* 31:149, 1985.

Reinecke RD: Ophthalmic examination of infants and children by the pediatrician. *Ped Clin N Amer* 30(6):995, 1983.

Sapira JD: An internist looks at the fundus oculi. *DM: Disease a Month* 30(14):1, 1984.

Walsh JB: Hypertensive retinopathy: Description, classification and prognosis. *Ophthalmology* 89:1127, 1982.

Whitman J, Cunningham RD: The red eye: Why it happens, what to do, when to refer. *Postgrad Med* 74(5):65, 1983.

chapter 7

Ear Procedures

EQUIPMENT AND SUPPLIES

Plastic aprons are worn by patients and staff during ear irrigation because of the high risk of soiling clothing.

A sharply focused light source is essential to good visualization of the ear. The classical head mirror works very well once one becomes familiar with its use. For a light source, use a standard focused examining lamp placed behind and to one side of the patient (figure 7-1). Alternatively, a head-mounted focusing operating light can be used.

A source of suction is desirable. Use a Baron or similar tip with a thumb-operated relief valve.

Other needed equipment includes emesis basins, bayonet or angled dressing forceps, Noyes or similar sturdy forceps for grasping foreign bodies, Goldnamer ear irrigating basin, a set of Brown or Gruber oval ear specula, malleable metal applicators to be used with cotton batting, Buck or similar ear curettes, a large ear syringe or pulsating water jet pump, and a standard otoscope with bulb for pneumatic otoscopy.

Required supplies include unsterile 4- by 4-inch gauze squares, facial

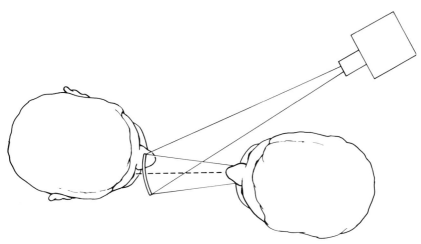

FIGURE 7-1
Use of the head mirror.

tissue, cotton balls, and perhaps some cylindrical cotton pledgets. Needed drugs include epinephrine 1:1000, tetracaine 2% solution or other topical anesthetic, and silver nitrate sticks. Cerumenex is a good agent for softening earwax if used properly as described below.

CERUMEN REMOVAL

Indications and technique of earwax removal vary with the patient's age and medical history. The most frequent indication in children is the need to see the eardrum to diagnose middle ear disease. Sometimes the ear(s) of a patient with external otitis need to be cleaned so that eardrops can reach the infected area. Wax is sometimes removed in an attempt to improve hearing; the benefits are small numerically but may be worth the effort in patients with significant hearing impairment. Some adults report dizziness or a pressure sensation in their ears which is relieved by removing plugs of wax. The author confesses that he cannot tell by inspection alone which wax accumulations represent significant "impacted cerumen" and which do not. The differentiation is made by asking how the patient feels before and after the procedure is done.

Cerumen may be removed by syringing or curetting. The former can be done either by a physician or a well-trained aide. The latter should be performed by a physician. Syringing carries risks of perforating the tympanic membrane or of contaminating the middle ear if there is a preexisting perforation or if tympanostomy tubes are in place. Normal intact eardrums are seldom damaged by proper syringing, but thin reparative membranes may perforate. Therefore the procedure should not be done on patients with a history of multiple previous episodes of otitis media unless the condition of the drums is known from previous examinations. It is also contraindicated in those wearing tympanostomy tubes.

Ear Syringing

Obtain appropriate historical information, and examine the ears to estimate the amount and condition of the cerumen. If it looks dark and hard, suggesting that it will resist being washed out, consider instilling some drops to soften it. Many different agents will soften earwax over a period of a few days: hydrogen peroxide solution, olive oil, docusate sodium, glycerol, mineral oil, and others. For faster results use triethanolamine polypeptide oleate condensate (Cerumenex), which will usually do the job in fifteen to thirty minutes. This product may cause irritation, especially if it is not syringed out promptly; consult manufacturer's literature before using it.

Have the patient tilt his or her head laterally so the drops can be instilled without contaminating the dropper tip. Put a plug of cotton in the ear loosely to catch any that may run out. Repeat the procedure on the opposite ear if indicated. While the drops are working, prepare a large basin of water, as close to body temperature as practical. Add a small amount of liquid soap. Position the patient in an ENT chair or on an examining table with the back raised almost to the vertical position. Both the patient and the operator should wear plastic aprons.

Hold the basin against the skin just below the ear to catch the water as it drains out. Check the axis of the ear canal before starting to irrigate, and direct the stream so that it flows along the roof of the canal in a effort to get it to flow past the plug and push it out from behind. The ear canal is sensitive; be careful not to scratch it with the instrument tip, and above all do not push cerumen or the instrument against the eardrum. Stop the procedure at intervals to monitor your results. If the plug becomes partly dislodged, you may be able to grasp it with thumb forceps or tease it out with a cotton-tip applicator.

CURETTING CERUMEN

This procedure requires firm immobilization. It may be done in either the sitting position or with the patient lying so that the ear to be treated is uppermost. Small children may be treated on the parent's lap, with one arm around the child's trunk and the other holding the patient's head firmly against the parent's chest. Pull the auricle posteriorly (in a child) or vertically (in an adult) to straighten the ear canal. If this procedure does not provide adequate visualization, use an oval ear speculum. Try to tease the mass free of the canal epithelium, and roll it out of the canal. In some cases it will be necessary to break up the mass and extract it in pieces. The ability to do this without traumatizing the skin and hurting the patient is a test of one's patience and dexterity.

FOREIGN BODY REMOVAL

Preschool children frequently insert foreign bodies into their ears, and insects may enter the ear canals of patients of all ages. Depending on the size and nature of the object, one or another of the following methods maybe used to remove them:

1. If the object is loose and not likely to swell if it becomes wet, wash it out with an ear syringe.

2. If it can be grasped easily, pull it out with a curette, hook, or forceps. Suitable hooks can often be improvised from paper clips.

3. Soft-tip tubes connected to vacuum pumps can be used to pull smooth objects out of the ear. Place the tube against the foreign body before turning on the suction.

4. Extremely strong cyanoacrylate glue (Super Glue, other brands) has reportedly been effective in removing hard objects. Straighten out a paper clip, wet the end of it with the glue, quickly touch it to the object for a minute or so until it sets, and pull gently. Do not use enough glue to form a drop; the excess is not needed and is likely to be lost in the canal.

5. The use of lidocaine spray has been advocated to stimulate a live insect to depart from the ear canal. If this fails, try the more traditional approach of drowning the creature by instilling mineral oil, ether, or other liquid and then removing it by one of the methods described above.

These procedures call for skill in gaining patient cooperation as well as manual gentleness and dexterity. Since small children tend to become combative when they are hurt, try to remove the object on the first maneuver. You may not get a second chance.

The methods described above may fail for many reasons. The patient may be too young or too frightened to hold still. An organic object such as a bean may swell after it gets into the ear canal. There may be an inflammatory reaction with epithelial edema. Removal under general anesthesia is required in such instances, both for pain control and also because motion of the head during instrumentation could cause the object to be driven through the tympanic membrane with disastrous results.

AURICULAR HEMATOMA

Blows or shearing forces to the auricle, most often seen in contact sports such as wrestling, may cause a hematoma to form between the ear cartilage and the overlying skin. If untreated, these lesions may become infected and may develop unsightly residual fibrosis ("cauliflower ear"). It is possible to temporize by emptying a hematoma with a syringe and large-bore needle, but surgical drainage is preferable because incompletely drained hematomas tend to recur.

Strict aseptic procedure is required because of the vulnerability of cartilage to infection. After scrubbing, draping, and injection of a local anesthetic agent without epinephrine, make a short incision over the most caudad portion of the hematoma. Express the blood, and insert a small

soft rubber drain. The dressing must provide gentle, even pressure, firm enough to encourage reapproximation of skin and cartilage but not enough to permit pressure necrosis. Cut gauze squares to shape to build up a dressing that will support the ear both medially and laterally, and then apply a circumferential pressure dressing, snug but not too tight. Remove the drain in two or three days.

Antibiotic therapy should be timed as for high-risk elective surgery: Give at least one dose before surgery, and discontinue the drug after the drain is removed.

HEARING TESTING

There is a hierarchy of techniques for hearing testing ranging from those that are inexpensive, simple, and inexact to those that involve significant costs, require some technical expertise, and give relatively precise results. Each has its place. Simple observation of a patient's inability to converse with you is an important functional test. If you think the person may be reading your lips, ask a question when he or she can't see your face. The value of listening for the ticking of a watch has diminished in the age of electronics, but you can rub your thumb and forefinger together an inch away from the patient's ear or use tuning forks to compare the patient's hearing with your own. The most useful forks for hearing testing are the 256-, 512-, and 1024-Hz instruments. Those of lower frequency measure primarily vibratory sense.

If you need to mask hearing with one ear while testing the other, put your index finger on the tragus of one ear and rub up and down as you test the other side.

A screening audiometer, built into an otoscope, is available from Welch Allyn Company. It gives useful screening data, but abnormal reports should be confirmed with more complete audiometric testing.

Pure-tone audiometers are relatively inexpensive, and it isn't difficult to learn to use them. However, the accuracy of the results obtained is strongly dependent on the level of background noise. Readings obtained in a relatively quiet examining room may be useful in detecting significant hearing losses or evaluating the results of treatment for otitis media, but legally valid audiograms require the use of a soundproof booth.

To perform an audiogram, first explain the procedure to the patient: He or she is to listen intently and raise a hand as a signal whenever hearing a musical sound, no matter whether it is high- or low-pitched, loud or soft. Put the earphones on yourself, and check that the instrument is working properly. Then place them on the patient; glasses and earrings should be removed and long hair pulled back since they may interfere with a snug fit between earphones and skin. Patients should be positioned so that you can see them easily but they cannot see your hands operating the audiometer. Start at one end of the frequency scale and a moderately loud (about 40 dB) tone. After the patient raises a hand to acknowledge hearing the tone, repeat the process at lower volumes until it can no longer be heard. Record the lowest intensity at which the sound is heard, and then repeat the process at the next frequency on the scale. When a complete curve has been obtained for one ear, do the same procedure on the other side. Plot the findings on a standard audiometric chart, using different symbols for the two ears.

Sound intensity is measured in decibels (dB), a logarithmic unit of sound in which 0 dB corresponds to the approximate hearing threshold of normal subjects. Each 10-dB change represents doubling of the sound intensity. Normal subjects often show test results of 15 dB, and occasionally up to 25 dB. Patients with 25- to 40-dB losses will have difficulty hearing faint speech, and those above 40 dB will have more severe hearing impairment. Inconsistent results may mean that the patient does not understand the test, is distracted, or is not cooperating fully. Repeat the procedure, mixing up frequencies and intensities, until you have obtained consistent results. An occasional patient will raise a hand at intervals whether or not hearing a sound. This problem is addressed by changing the cadence of the test sounds and encouraging the person not to raise a hand unless certain of hearing something.

SUGGESTED READING

Das SK: Aetiological evaluation of foreign bodies in the ear and nose. *J Laryngol Otol* 98:989, 1984.

Gershel J, Kruger B, Giraudi-Perry D, et al: Accuracy of the Welch Allyn AudioScope and traditional hearing screening for children with known hearing loss. *J Pediat* 106:15, 1985.

McDermott JC, Giebink S, Le CT, et al: Children with persistent otitis media: Audiometric and tympanometric findings. *Arch Otolaryngol* 109:360, 1983.

Olsen WO: Presbycusis: When hearing wanes, is amplification the answer? *Postgrad Med* 76(3):189, 1984.

Snyder J: Office audiometry. *J Fam Pract* 19:535, 1984.

chapter 8

Nose Procedures

EQUIPMENT AND SUPPLIES

Plastic aprons are worn by patients and staff during treatment of nosebleeds because of the high risk that splattered blood will soil clothing.

As with ear procedures a sharply focused light source is essential to good visualization of the nose. The classical head mirror is once again recommended, as is a standard-focused examining lamp placed behind and to one side of the patient. Alternatively, a head-mounted focusing operating light can be used.

A source of suction is needed. Use a small suction tip with thumb-operated relief valve.

Also needed are emesis basins, bayonet or angulated dressing forceps, and bivalve nasal specula.

Required supplies include unsterile 4- by 4-inch gauze squares, facial tissue, and cotton balls or cylindrical pledgets. Needed drugs include epinephrine 1:1000, tetracaine 2% solution or other topical anesthetic, and silver nitrate sticks. A 4% cocaine solution is a very effective vasoconstrictor and topical anesthetic which may be stocked if security is not a problem. However, cocaine is potentially toxic; use only the amount that can be held by one cotton pledget, well wrung out.

CLINICAL EXAMINATION

Nasal examination and treatment are best done with the patient sitting and the head supported. This is easiest to accomplish with an ENT chair, but a reasonable approximation can be obtained by lifting the back of a standard examining table almost to the vertical position. Otoscopes permit only limited inspection of the nose; a head-mounted light or the traditional head mirror doesn't get in the doctor's way, gives brighter light, and affords excellent visualization of the nose and other cavities. Use a standard bivalve nasal speculum, held so that the blades push upward and downward, not laterally.

EPISTAXIS

Physicians in primary care see numerous patients with bleeding noses, almost all of them originating in Kiesselbach's plexus on the anterior part of the septum. Since you are unlikely to encounter other types frequently enough to develop proficiency in their treatment, it makes sense to become proficient in the management of anterior epistaxis and refer other types to an ENT specialist.

Nosebleeds often occur in association with upper respiratory infections, dryness of the air, and minor trauma. Repeated episodes may occur from a single tiny bleeding point. Since there is a small possibility that the problem is a manifestation of a bleeding disorder or other systemic disease, it is important to obtain a brief medical history before treatment is started. How long has the patient been bleeding? Is this a new problem or a recurrent one? Is there a history of abnormal bleeding in the patient or close relatives? Does the patient have other health problems or take drugs that might contribute to the problem? Any associated dizziness, nausea, or other symptoms?

Record the patient's blood pressure and pulse at intervals. High blood pressure readings may reflect either true hypertension or anxiety about the epistaxis. Abnormally low readings may reflect significant blood loss.

Position the patient and light source, and inspect the nose. Have the patient blow his or her nose to clear as much of the blood and clots as possible, and then clean out the remainder, either with suction or with the judicious use of thumb forceps and applicators. Locate the bleeding point; if it isn't on the anterior nasal septum (Kiesselbach's area) and the patient is still bleeding actively, consider immediate ENT referral.

The next step in managing the typical anterior nosebleed is to try to stop it with a combination of vasoconstriction and direct pressure. Use a cotton pledget or draw a cotton ball out into a cylindrical shape, the diameter of a pencil and an inch or more in length. Soak it with 1:1000 epinephrine or 4% cocaine. Use thumb forceps to place it in the nostril against the bleeding point. Have the patient apply steady, continuous pressure laterally against the nose to compress the cotton pledget against the septum (figure 8-1). Pinching both nostrils forces the patient to mouth-breathe and is not necessary to control the bleeding.

After about ten minutes, remove the cotton and check to see if the bleeding has stopped. If it has, cauterize the area with a silver nitrate stick to discourage recurrence. If it has not, apply the silver nitrate anyhow in an attempt to stop the flow of blood. Electrocautery may also be used, but only after a topical anesthetic such as tetracaine or cocaine has been applied.

Authorities differ as to whether the nose should be packed after

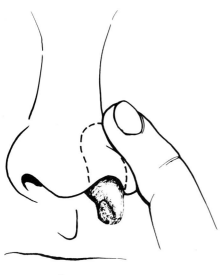

FIGURE 8-1
Controlling anterior nose bleed.

bleeding stops. The author prefers to insert a second pledget, wetted with 1:1000 epinephrine, and instruct the patient or family to leave it in place at least overnight. Use paper adhesive tape to hold it in place, but do not block the opposite nostril.

Patients can often manage nosebleeds at home in a similar manner. A cotton ball or rolled-up segment of facial tissue can be moistened with water or nasal decongestant solution and inserted into the nostril, after which steady, lateral pressure is applied to the nose for ten minutes or longer. The plug should be taped in place until the next day. If the problem recurs, you may wish to have the patient come in for cautery. Be prepared for bleeding to start when the scab over the previous bleeding point is disturbed.

Finding a purulent discharge associated with nasal bleeding in a child should lead you to look for a foreign body.

FOREIGN BODIES

Small children frequently insert pebbles and other foreign objects into their nostrils, where they act as foreign bodies inducing edema and a purulent discharge. Their removal may be simple if the problem is approached methodically, but general anesthesia may be required if the child is unable to cooperate or if the object is unusually difficult to dislodge.

Start by applying vasoconstrictor drops in the nostril to reduce edema.

A 2% ephedrine solution has been recommended, but xylometazoline is more widely available and should be satisfactory. Wait ten minutes before proceeding.

In some instances the child can, with instruction, blow the object out. Have the child close his or her mouth and occlude the opposite nostril. There are reports in the literature of physicians accomplishing the same thing in a procedure similar to mouth-to-mouth resuscitation: You block the opposite nostril with finger pressure, breathe into the child's mouth until increasing pressure is felt, and then exhale sharply to blow the object out.

If these measures fail and the child can hold still, you may be able to remove the object with forceps or a hook improvised from a paper clip. Be careful not to push the object backward since it could be aspirated from the throat into the lungs. Removal of large soft objects can sometimes be made easier by cutting them in half with small scissors. As a last resort, arrange for removal under general anesthesia.

When you find one foreign body, look for others in the same and opposite nostrils.

SUGGESTED READING

Guazzo E: Removal of foreign bodies from the nose (letter). *N Engl J Med* 312:725, 1985.

Myer CM, Cotton RT: Nasal obstruction in the pediatric patient. *Pediatrics* 72:766, 1983.

chapter 9

Pharynx and Larynx

EQUIPMENT

The head mirror and light source described in chapter 7 can also be used, with a laryngeal mirror, to examine the hypopharynx and larynx. Alternatively, a small lighted right-angle laryngeal telescope may be employed. A long curved forceps is needed for removal of pharyngeal foreign bodies.

INDIRECT LARYNGOSCOPY

Visualization of the hypopharynx and larynx with a laryngeal mirror is a skill that comes only with practice (figure 9-1). Its principal indication in primary care is to inspect the vocal cords of hoarse patients. It is also useful for removing fishbones and other sharp foreign bodies from the hypopharynx.

If the patient can relax and cooperate fully, the procedure will usually go quickly. Some patients are more susceptible than others to gagging, but it is more likely to be a problem in those who become tense. Once gagging starts, it is difficult to stop. To minimize this problem, instruct the patient to breathe freely through the mouth. Do not let the mirror touch the posterior third of the tongue or the wall of the pharynx. Experienced examiners can usually perform the procedure without anesthesia, but if gagging becomes a problem or seems likely to, anesthetize the pharynx and posterior tongue by spraying a topical anesthetic such as 2% tetracaine solution. Explain to the patient that you plan to numb the throat to diminish the normal gag reflex but that the anesthetic solution should not be inhaled or swallowed. As you depress the tongue with a tongue depressor, instruct the patient to take in a deep breath and then exhale slowly, saying "eee" as you spray. Give the patient a kidney basin into which to expectorate, and have a supply of tissues or gauze squares at hand.

Since the patient's exhaled breath is warm and humid, the mirror will tend to fog. This can be prevented in one of three ways:

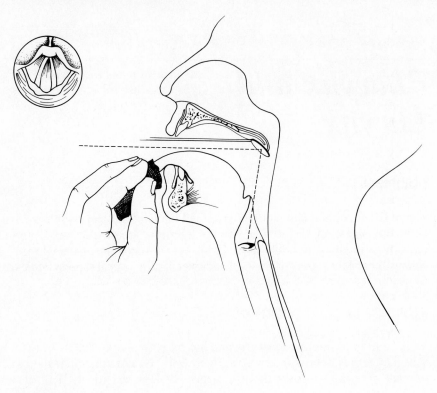

FIGURE 9-1
Indirect laryngoscopy.

1. Keep a basin of warm water at hand to warm the mirror. Wipe water droplets off with a gauze square before use.
2. Warm the mirror with a small flame, as from an alcohol lamp. Touch the instrument to the back of your hand each time before inserting it in the patient's mouth to be sure it is not warm enough to cause a burn.
3. Use a proprietary anti-fog spray.

Position the patient in a seated position, leaning forward with the head extended into a slightly chin-up position. Any dentures should be removed. Adjust your head mirror or lamp so that the light will strike the mirror as it is advanced. ENT specialists often prefer to hold the patient's tongue with their nondominant hand, but those who do the procedure less often may prefer to let the patient do the holding. Give the patient a 4-inch gauze square to use to grasp the tongue. The person should pull it as far forward as possible with comfort, although avoiding an excess of force that could stimulate the gag reflex. Hold the mirror in your dominant hand as you would a pen. The heel of your hand may rest against the patient's cheek to aid stability.

Use a #4- or #5-size mirror unless there is a specific need for a smaller one. After warming the mirror or applying an antifog solution, advance it carefully through the open mouth until it rests against and slightly indents the soft palate and uvula. Move smoothly and confidently to minimize shaking that could stimulate the gag reflex. Touching the palate usually causes no problems. The handle of the mirror is malleable and can be bent slightly if needed for a particular patient. Inspect the hypopharynx as it comes into view and then the larynx. Then have the patient take a deep breath and slowly exhale, saying "heeee" at a high, falsetto pitch to facilitate inspection of the vocal cords. Demonstrate the sound you want. Watch the motion of the cords; they should come together smoothly for phonation and spring apart symmetrically during inspiration.

Lighted right-angle telescopes designed for laryngoscopy are more costly than laryngeal mirrors but are relatively easy to use and are well tolerated by patients. The procedure is essentially the same as for mirror examination. Use an antifog solution on the objective lens surface.

PHARYNGEAL FOREIGN BODIES

Small, sharp foreign bodies occasionally become lodged in the throat. Possible sites include the tonsil, base of the tongue, one of the valleculae or pyriform fossae, or the postcricoid region. An object embedded in a tonsil can be removed with forceps. One which has lodged in the vallecula or other part of the hypopharynx can be visualized with a laryngeal mirror and removed with a large curved foreign body forceps or surgical clamp. Sometimes nothing abnormal can be found on examination of a patient who complains of a foreign body sensation; this may indicate local abrasion caused by a sharp object which subsequently passed on through the enteric tract. However, it could also indicate that the foreign body became embedded in the tissues or lodged in the esophagus. X-rays and/or ENT consultation is required unless there is prompt, spontaneous resolution of the symptoms.

SUGGESTED READING

Deweese DD, Saunders WH: *Textbook of Otolaryngology,* 5th ed. St. Louis, Mosby, 1977.

chapter 10

Spirometry

Spirometry is the measurement of airflow into and out of the lungs for the purpose of diagnosing pulmonary (and occasionally extrapulmonary) disease and for assessing changes therein over time. These changes may be spontaneous or in response to treatment. Spirometry is a sensitive, essentially noninvasive, and relatively inexpensive tool which has many uses in primary care.

Pulmonary disease specialists have devised complex terminology and methods of measurement, but the primary physician needs to be conversant with only selected parts of this technology. Office spirometry measures the two or three parameters most likely to indicate disorders of airflow. Normal test results usually do not require external confirmation if they are consistent with the clinical picture. Abnormal findings often represent an indication for referring the patient for more specialized and detailed pulmonary function testing.

Planning for office spirometry involves a number of interrelated considerations: What kinds of patients will be tested, and with what objectives? How much expenditure for equipment is justifiable considering anticipated patient volume and reimbursement? What personnel are available to perform the tests, and who will train them? Who will oversee the quality of the testing done? Has a firm and unequivocal commitment been made that the spirometry will be of consistently unimpeachable quality?

The quality issue is important. Spirometry is not like electrocardiography, where technical errors are usually evident on the tracing. Many spirometric mistakes can go unrecognized to the detriment of patient care, so it is essential that personnel be both highly motivated and well trained. Even with the best of training, though, abnormal results must not be accepted uncritically. Clinical correlation is essential, and confirmation from a reliable pulmonary function laboratory may be indicated. Periodic maintenance and calibration are required; their nature and extent will vary with the type of instrument.

Office spirometry does not require the precision of that done for research purposes, but the technique must be consistent so that repeat determinations over time are closely comparable.

Training of personnel can sometimes be conducted by the vendor; determine the qualifications and willingness to provide this service at the time the purchase or lease is being negotiated. In some cases local hospital personnel will be willing to do the necessary training. It does not require a great amount of time, but it must be done correctly.

INDICATIONS FOR SPIROMETRY

1. Workup of the dyspneic patient. The most common diagnoses in this category are asthma and chronic obstructive pulmonary disease (COPD). Restrictive lung diseases such as pulmonary fibrosis and sarcoidosis may also be seen from time to time. Left-sided congestive heart failure may cause spirometric abnormalities which usually clear when the underlying process is controlled. In some instances the diagnosis of psychogenic dyspnea can be assisted by spirometry.
2. Monitoring response to treatment. The frequent use of spirometry at home has been advocated as an adjunct to the management of difficult asthma patients; for this purpose simple peak-flow meters will suffice. Serial office measurements are useful in monitoring the course of other chronic pulmonary disease processes.
3. Baseline measurements and periodic follow-up of patients at high risk for development of pulmonary diseases, including smokers and people exposed to industrial pulmonary irritants.
4. Part of the evaluation of persons claiming pulmonary disability. These people will require spirometry that meets the requirements of agencies such as the Occupational Safety and Health Administration.
5. Evaluation of pulmonary disease patients anticipating elective surgery.

EQUIPMENT

Spirometers for office use are of two general types: Those that measure the volume of air in an expansible container at any moment and plot changes in this volume over time, and those that measure airflow (pneumotach instruments). Many of the latter are equipped to compute volume changes electronically. Volume spirometers are of three types: Those that have a chamber that moves up and down in a container of water, those with a rolling sealing system, and those operating on a bellows principle. The "wet" systems are seldom seen in primary care settings. Bellows instruments are often rudimentary and inexpensive but quite adequate for screening purposes.

Some inexpensive flow-measuring spirometers are driven by small internal turbine wheels which rotate in response to air movement; they typically measure only peak airflow rates and are used chiefly to guide the management of asthma patients. Newer computerized flow-measuring instruments are relatively expensive but, because of their sophisticated circuitry, can create elaborate printouts of multiple pulmonary function parameters.

CLINICAL MEASUREMENT OF RESPIRATORY AIR FLOW

The normal flow of air in the resting subject is spoken of as the *tidal volume* (TV). The additional amount which a subject can forcefully inhale over and above the tidal volume is called the *inspiratory reserve volume* (IRV). The volume which can be exhaled from the resting position is spoken of as the *expiratory reserve volume* (ERV). The sum of these three, the total amount one can forcefully exhale after taking in as large a breath as possible, is called the *forced vital capacity* (FVC). The FVC is reduced in various forms of restrictive pulmonary disease and in the pulmonary congestion associated with left-heart failure.

The rate at which the lungs can be emptied of air is a useful measure of obstructive pulmonary diseases, most commonly asthma or COPD. The easiest and most often used way to evaluate this is to measure what fraction of the FVC is exhaled in one second (*forced expiratory volume, one second,* or FEV_1). In the early stages of COPD flow rates tend to decrease while volume remains relatively normal. Later both may be impaired.

An alternative measure of expiratory flow rate is called the *forced expiratory flow from 25 to 75 percent* (FEF 25–75%). It was formerly called the *maximal midexpiratory flow rate* (MMEFR). It is calculated by setting a point on the expiratory flow curve 25 percent of the volume down from full inspiration, setting another on the curve 75 percent of the way down, connecting the two points with a straight line, and calculating the corresponding flow velocity. This measurement is said by some writers to be more sensitive than the FEV_1/FVC to the small airway abnormality associated with chronic smoking, but others feel that the results may be misleading.

In spirometric testing, the patient is connected to the machine through a mouthpiece, takes a maximal breath in, and then empties the lungs forcefully and completely as a timed volume tracing is made. All three of the above parameters can be calculated from a single tracing.

TECHNIQUE

Pertinent patient data are recorded; these include name, chart number, date and time of examination, sex, age, height, weight, and the presence of any significant physical abnormalities such as kyphoscoliosis. For patients with orthopedic disorders which preclude measuring the height, an approximation can be obtained from the arm span.

Authorities differ as to whether the patient should be standing or sitting. The expected measurement differences aren't great, but testing should be done consistently in one position or the other. All tight clothing, including brassieres and girdles, should be loosened. Dentures are removed. The procedure is explained to the patient, and the technician demonstrates the method personally. A disposable mouthpiece attached to the equipment is placed in the patient's mouth and gripped by the teeth or gums, with the lips closed tight. A clip is placed to close off the nose. After having had a few seconds to relax and breathe normally through the machine the patient is instructed to take as deep a breath as possible and then forcefully blow it out. Exhalation is continued until the line is flat, usually requiring four to six seconds. When no more air can be expelled, the patient is permitted to resume normal breathing. The process is repeated until at least three technically satisfactory tracings have been acquired. At this point the patient is disconnected from the spirometer. It should be flushed out with fresh air between tests if it is of the volume type.

The key to accurate, reliable testing is motivating the patient to take truly maximal efforts to inspire and expire fully. This requires shouting at the patient: "Blow! Blow! That's it! Harder! Harder! Keep going! More! More!" Only if the patient becomes truly hypoxemic should the procedure be discontinued prematurely.

Figure 10-1 illustrates the type of tracing obtained. The initial upward curve represents a resting respiratory cycle. The larger rise which follows represents voluntary maximal inspiration. This is followed by forced expiration, rapidly at first and then more slowly until as much air as possible has been blown out. About four seconds after this phase was initiated, the subject is permitted to resume normal breathing. The various volume parameters which can be measured from this type of tracing (IRV, TV, ERV, and FEV_1) are illustrated, along with the slope of the line for determining FEF 25–75%. Plastic overlays for determining the latter without calculation are supplied by the instrument manufacturers.

On research spirometric equipment and on the illustrations in this chapter, the line moves upward as the patient inhales and downward with expiration. In many clinical spirometers the movement is in the opposite direction, with the line rising as the patient exhales. Either way, the curves should be fair, with no evidence of hesitation by the patient or mechanical resistance to airflow.

Since expired air is at body temperature and saturated with water vapor (BTPS conditions), and therefore of different density from room air, a

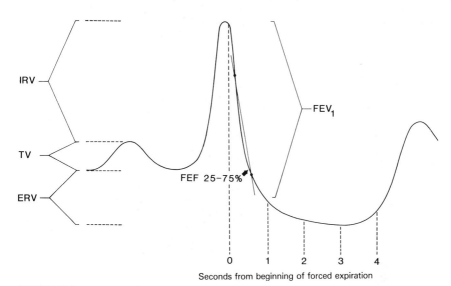

FIGURE 10-1
Spirometric tracing.

correction factor must be applied to the volume measurements. The method for doing this varies from one machine to another.

The zero point for measuring the onset of forced expiration is inherently somewhat imprecise, so an arbitrary process called *back extrapolation* is used to set it (figure 10-2). Draw two lines on the paper over the test tracing, one along the steepest part of the expiration curve and the other horizontally from the point of deepest inspiration. The point where these lines intersect is arbitrarily called the *zero time point*. To ensure that the point is meaningful and the test technically satisfactory, draw a vertical line segment from the zero point to the expiration curve. The

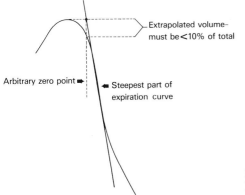

FIGURE 10-2
Back extrapolation.

length of this segment should represent no more than 10 percent of the total expired volume. This calculation is done automatically by many microprocessor-controlled spirometers.

The technician should make a note with regard to the patient's level of cooperation and an estimate of the reliability of the test results.

Standards for patients of varying age, height, and sex have been published in tabular and nomogram form (see this chapter's "Suggested Reading" and manufacturers literature). However, they do not adequately address other variables such as race and socioeconomic status. There is difference of opinion about cutoff points between normal and abnormal values; 20 percent variation from statistical norms is usually considered evidence of disease, but narrower limits of normality may be established in time.

TESTING BEFORE AND AFTER BRONCHODILATORS

It is often helpful to test patients before and after the use of bronchodilator drugs, both to diagnose the presence of reversible bronchospasm and to evaluate response to prescribed bronchodilators. Different authorities favor different drugs for this purpose. One protocol is to use two inhalations of isoetharine from a metered-dose inhaler during a single slow inspiration. Isoproterenol and metaproterenol have also been recommended for this purpose, although there is some disagreement about the appropriate doses. A range of 0.65 to 2.60 mg of metaproterenol (one to four inhalations from a metered-dose inhaler or its equivalent from a hand-held nebulizer) has been suggested. The postbronchodilator testing should be timed to concide with the peak effect of the drug (for metaproterenol, ten to forty-five minutes after administration). A significant positive response to this procedure is indicated by an increase in FVC on the order of 15 percent or more, increase in FEV_1 of 12 percent or more, and increase in FEF 25–75% of 45 percent or more. In this context it is more reliable to compare absolute changes in FEV_1 rather than changes in the FEV_1/FVC ratio.

PITFALLS AND SOURCES OF ERROR

1. Air leak at the mouth or nose, or in the equipment
2. A tense patient
3. Incomplete emptying of the lungs
4. Hesitation at the beginning of expiration
5. Failure to correct for temperature and humidity

6. Recent exposure to inhalants and/or drugs which may affect test results in either direction
7. Machine malfunctioning
8. Failure to calibrate the machine as often as required
9. Overinterpretation of test results, and failure to correlate them with the total clinical picture

SUGGESTED READING

Conrad SA, Kinasewitz GT, George RB (eds): *Pulmonary Function Testing: Principles and Practice.* New York, Churchill Livingstone, 1984.

Crapo RO, Morris AH, Gardner RM: Reference spirometric values using techniques and equipment that meets ATS recommendations. *Am Rev Respir Dis* 123:659, 1981.

Butler J: The pulmonary function test: Cautious overinterpretation. *Chest* 79:498, 1981.

Eichenhorn MS, Beauchamp R, Harper PA, et al: An assessment of three portable peak flow meters. *Chest* 82:306,1982.

Katz DN: The Mini-Wright peak flow meter for evaluating airway obstruction in a family practice. *J Fam Pract* 17:51, 1983.

Petty TL: Spirometry in clinical practice. *Postgrad Med* 69(4):122, 1981.

Ruppel G: *Manual of Pulmonary Function Testing,* 3d ed. St. Louis, Mosby, 1982.

Section on Respiratory Pathophysiology: Statement on spirometry. *Chest* 83:547, 1983.

Wall MA: Office pulmonary function testing. *Ped Clin N Amer* 31(4):773, 1984.

Wilson AF (ed): *Pulmonary Function Testing: Indications and Interpretations.* Orlando, Fla., Grune & Stratton, 1985.

chapter 11

Electrocardiography

Consultant: MICHAEL D. SCHAEN, M.D.

The material in this section will be familiar to physicians. It is written for the benefit of staff members who take electrocardiograms.

The heart is a muscular organ about the size of one's fist which contains four chambers and four valves. It contracts rhythmically, pumping blood through the arteries to all parts of the body. Every time a heart muscle fiber contracts, it generates a very small electrical force. All the fibers in the heart beating together create roughly one-hundredth volt or one ten-thousandth of the strength of household electrical supply. The electrocardiograph (often abbreviated ECG or EKG) is a sensitive machine which detects this current and traces it on a moving sheet of paper. The general configuration and system of naming different parts of the tracing are illustrated in figure 11-1, which shows two beats with a standardization mark after the second one.

The first deflection, caused by contraction of the small upper chambers of the heart, is arbitrarily named the *P wave.* The next part, caused by contraction of the thick-walled lower chambers (ventricles), is called the *QRS complex;* the initial downward deflection is named *Q,* the upward movement is designated *R,* and the final downward part is called *S.* The final deflection, the *T wave,* is caused by the myocardial fibers getting ready to beat again.

The different components have different configurations in different "leads" of the electrocardiogram. By connecting multiple electrodes to different parts of the patient and switching among them, the heart's

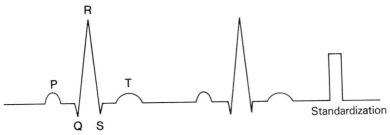

FIGURE 11-1
Electrocardiographic tracing.

functioning is measured from different angles. This switching must be done manually on older machines, but newer ones do it automatically.

The electrocardiogram (electrocardiographic tracing) can give information about the heart's rhythm. Some irregularities are worrisome but others are insignificant. Many occur intermittently and therefore may be missed on a single tracing. The ECG is also a valuable tool in the diagnosis of both recent (acute) and long-standing (chronic) diseases of the heart muscle. The most common type is coronary artery disease, or blockage of one or more of the small arteries which supply nourishment to the heart muscle itself. Chest pain has many causes, of which coronary artery disease is only one. The ECG is often helpful in determining the cause in a particular patient. The test measures voltage and does nothing more; *patients can be assured that it will not harm them in any way.*

The paper on which ECG tracings are recorded is printed in a grid pattern, the fine lines 1 mm apart and the heavy lines 5 mm apart. The usual paper speed is 25 mm per second, corresponding to 25 fine lines or 5 heavy ones. Thus the interval between fine lines is 0.04 second, and that between heavy lines is 0.2 second. Most machines can also record at double speed, 50 mm per second, for special purposes. The vertical deflection is normally one millivolt (mV) per millimeter; some machines can be set for greater or lesser sensitivity. Electrocardiograph machines contain internal voltage standards of 10 mV which are used to be sure the sensitivity of the equipment is properly set. A 10-mV mark should appear on each segment of the tracing. It will be put on automatically by newer equipment; the method of making standardization marks with older ECG machines is described below.

There are twelve standard "leads," each representing a different combination of electrodes and therefore recording the heart's electrical activity in a different dimension. They are recorded and printed out in a standardized sequence. The first six, called I, II, III, aVR, aVL, and aVF, respectively, are made by switching among the arm and leg electrodes. The second six are taken from a series of points on the chest wall and are labeled, in order, V_1 through V_6. Modern multichannel electrocardiographs also produce an extra length of lead II which is intended to facilitate the detection of irregular rhythms; it is called a *rhythm strip*.

TECHNIQUE

The patient will need to undress to the waist and have bare wrists and ankles. Heavy metal watches and jewelry are removed. Women are provided with a cape or short gown which may be moved aside while the chest electrodes are being applied. The procedure is normally done with the patient lying supine, although the head may be raised somewhat for comfort. Be sure the patient is relaxed and reasonably warm since shivering or other muscle contractions may appear as artifacts on the tracing.

Electrodes are marked to indicate the location where they are to be applied. Serious technical errors will occur if any are put in the wrong place. One electrode is applied to each wrist and each ankle, using the elastic band which is a part of the electrode. These bands should be snug enough for solid contact but not tight enough to cause discomfort, impede circulation, or cause artifacts on the tracing. An electrically conductive material, either disposable saturated pads or electrode paste, is applied between skin and electrodes to ensure perfect electrical contact. If the paste is used, it should be rubbed in well; it contains a mild abrasive agent to break through the relatively nonconductive outer layers of the skin.

Chest electrodes usually incorporate small suction cups for skin attachment. Newer systems which record all twelve leads automatically have six suction cups that are applied simultaneously, while older ones have a single electrode that must be moved between one V lead and the next. Some systems have a broad weighted rubber sash which is placed across the chest and used to hold a movable chest electrode in place. Apply the electrodes firmly to skin in the proper location using either disposable saturated pads or electrode paste to complete the contact. With suction electrodes, only the paste is satisfactory. If a woman's breast gets in the way, ask her to hold it up and to the side while you position the electrodes.

Positioning the six V leads requires some knowledge of the anatomy of the chest (figure 11-2). The sternum, or breastbone, runs vertically in the middle. The clavicles, or collarbones, start near the top of the sternum and run laterally to the shoulders. The ribs also run laterally from the sternum; the first pair are covered by the clavicles, so the first that can be felt are the second ribs (counting from top down). The spaces between the ribs, called interspaces, are numbered according to the rib just above; thus the fourth interspace is between the fourth and fifth ribs.

A series of imaginary lines are use to position the V leads laterally. The *midclavicular line* runs vertically down from the middle of the clavicle. The *anterior axillary* line runs straight downward from the anterior border of the axilla (armpit). The *midaxillary line* runs vertically from the middle of the axilla. The V leads are positioned as follows:

V_1—fourth interspace, just to (patient's) right of the sternum

V_2—fourth interspace, just to the left of the sternum

V_3—midway between V_2 and V_4

V_4—fifth interspace at midclavicular line

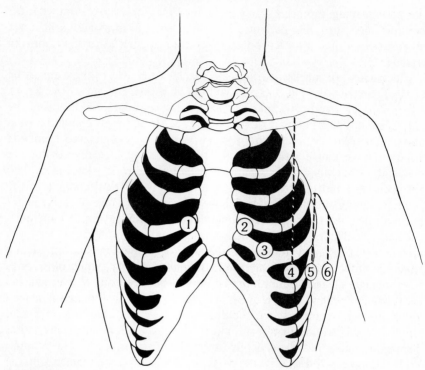

FIGURE 11-2
Positioning of chest electrodes.

V_5—anterior axillary line directly lateral from V_4
V_6—midaxillary line directly lateral from V_4.

Recording of the actual tracing is done at the push of a single button on many newer machines, with all twelve leads plus a rhythm strip being recorded and additional data printed out automatically. Older equipment requires more attention and dexterity: Turn the lead selector switch to each lead in turn. Turn the main switch on to the position in which the recording stylus moves but the paper remains stationary. Check to be sure the stylus is not bumping the top or bottom of its range, and center it manually (using the centering knob) if necessary. Then turn the switch to the recording position, and observe the tracing being recorded. Press the standardization button for a fraction of a second between beats to record the standardization voltage. Press the lead-marking button to indicate which lead is being recorded. Turn the machine off as soon as a sufficient length of tracing has been obtained (between three and six seconds, depending on the system used to mount the tracings). If there seems to be some abnormality, take an extra-long tracing and consult with the physician before cutting it down for mounting. Advance the lead selector switch to the next mark and repeat the sequence. For the V leads, set the switch and move the chest electrode between leads as described above. This sequence sounds complicated, but it can be mastered by practicing on a friend or coworker to become familiar with electrocardiographic technique and pertinent anatomic landmarks.

The lead-marking button makes a mark at the top of the recording paper as long as the button is held down. It permits marking of each segment of the tracing for precise identification. The following code may be used:

I	–	V_1	– .
II	– –	V_2	– . .
III	– – –	V_3	– . . .
aVR	. –	V_4	– . . . .
aVL	. . –	V_5	– . . . . .
aVF	. . . –	V_6	– . . . . . .

Errors caused by applying electrodes to the wrong arms or legs may be detected by checking the height of the R and S waves and using the following formulas as rough checks:

$$I + III = II$$

$$aVR + aVL + aVF = 0$$

If the date, time, and patient identification are not recorded automatically, write them on the tracing immediately. Then remove the electrodes, and wipe any electrode paste from the patient's skin with wet paper towels. Clean the contact surfaces well to ensure that they will always give good electrical conductance.

SUGGESTED READING

Lyon LJ: *Basic Electrocardiography Handbook.* New York, Van Nostrand Reinhold, 1977.

Marriott HJL: *Practical Electrocardiography,* 5th ed. Baltimore, Williams & Wilkins, 1972.

chapter 12

Female Reproductive Tract

Consultant: BRADLEY BUSACCO, M.D.

Well-done pelvic examinations and related laboratory procedures can provide much clinically useful information about infections, pregnancy, tumors, and other conditions of the female reproductive organs. Since this part of the body is endowed with both great physical sensitivity and major symbolic significance, gentleness, tact, and understanding on the part of the examiner are important. This topic is being addressed in greater detail than many other procedures because it is performed so frequently and because fine points of technique can have a major impact both on patient comfort and on the quantity and quality of information obtained from the examination.

EQUIPMENT AND SUPPLIES

The examining room should be comfortably warm and should offer both visual and auditory privacy. There should be a place for the patient to put clothing out of sight, either in a drawer or behind a screen. The examining table should be located so that the patient's perineum does not face the door.

Standard examining tables with retractable leg supports and stirrups are satisfactory. The patient is examined in lithotomy position with her hips at the edge of the table. Many patients will be more comfortable if the head of the table is raised a foot or so. This position also facilitates eye contact and dialogue between patient and examiner. Watching the patient's face will let you know immediately if any part of the procedure causes pain. Disposable paper draping sheets are widely used although they are stiffer than cloth and tend to slide out of position. This problem can be minimized by tucking the corners of the drape under the patient's hips. It's useful to have a small mirror available with which the patient can watch as various aspects of the procedure and findings are explained to her. A bright, suitably focused examining light is essential to the conduct of a proper pelvic examination. Many types are available, either freestanding or designed for wall or ceiling mounting. Some physicians favor an ENT examining light mounted on the examiner's head; although this approach has not been widely adopted, it has the advantage of providing well-focused light on the same axis as the examiner's eyes but with nothing that can get in the way of the hands. The traditional gooseneck lamp using standard household light bulbs is mentioned only to be condemned. It gets in the examiner's way, and if the bulb is powerful enough to provide adequate light, there is a risk of burning the patient's legs.

Vaginal specula of different sizes should be at hand to accommodate varying clinical needs. The appropriate size for a particular patient can usually be deduced from the sexual and obstetrical history. It may occasionally be necessary to try different sizes. If metal specula are used, they should be warmed to body temperature before use. Some examining tables have speculum storage drawers containing small electric heating elements to keep specula warm. Alternatively, you can run warm water over a speculum before insertion. This will warm it and lubricate it enough for most examining purposes. Reusable vaginal specula should be cleaned thoroughly and then autoclaved between uses. They need not be kept in sterile wraps. Disposable plastic specula are favored in some practices. They do not feel cold to touch, and they eliminate the need for washing and sterilization, but some physicians find them awkward to use. A detailed equipment and supply list is given in chapter 19, "Equipment and Supplies."

THE PELVIC EXAMINATION

Obtain your history before the patient undresses. The quality of the information you elicit will be higher than if you interviewed her on an examining table, and she will appreciate the opportunity to become acquainted with the examiner before submitting to the procedure. A chaperone should always be present when a pelvic examination is conducted by a male physician. This protects the physician against accusations of immoral behavior and also relieves the anxieties of patients, some of whom may experience a sense of physical vulnerability if a chaperone is not present. Female examiners do not require chaperones, but some prefer to have one present to get the patient ready, facilitate the handling of specimens, and help calm apprehensive patients.

Before the patient disrobes, ask her how recently she has urinated. If her bladder may be full enough to interfere with the examination, have her void. If urinalysis may be indicated, this is the time to get a specimen if it wasn't obtained earlier. Ask whether the patient has douched recently since this would wash away any vaginal secretions and could invalidate a significant part of the examination.

As a general principle, your stronger hand should be used to palpate the suprapubic area while your more sensitive hand does the internal examination. There is no firm rule on this, however. Indeed, some physicians prefer to examine the adnexal structures on one side with one hand, and then reglove and examine the opposite side with the other hand. The "inside" hand must be gloved, if only to protect the examiner from the occasional patient with unrecognized infection. Many physicians wear a glove on the other hand also. Disposable gloves that have not been sterilized are satisfactory unless the patient is pregnant near term.

Keep the patient informed at each stage of the procedure at a level consistent with her sophistication and interest. Some want to know more details than others. The examination starts with inspection of the perineum. Look for tumors, inflammation, excoriation, warts, ectoparasites, and anomalies. Then separate the labia gently, and inspect the vaginal and urethral orifices and clitoris. Ask the patient to bear down (Valsalva's maneuver), and inspect for cystocele, rectocele, and uterine prolapse.

The speculum examination is usually done before the digital exam because lubricants used on examining gloves may destroy specimens obtained for Papanicolaou tests. Sometimes it's better to do the digital examination first, particularly if it proves difficult to visualize the cervix through the speculum. The speculum examination is usually done with the examiner seated, and the bimanual portion standing up.

Since the long axis of the labia runs vertically there is a temptation to rotate the speculum 90 degrees so that its blades will more nearly conform to the configuration of the labia during insertion. However, the fibromuscular introitus is wider than it is high, so the patient will have less discomfort if you insert the speculum with the blades horizontal and the handle pointing downward. With obese patients it is sometimes helpful to turn the speculum so that the handle points upward. Gently spread the labia with two fingers of the "outside" hand to visualize the introitus (figure 12-1). Since the area around the urethral meatus is more sensitive than the posterior aspect of the introitus, it is better to introduce the speculum a bit too far posterior than too far anterior. If undue resistance to advancement is noted, use a smaller speculum. If redundant folds of vaginal mucosa make it difficult to visualize the cervix, use a larger one. Once the tip of the speculum is through the introitus, apply gentle pressure on the thumb lever of the speculum to spread the blades apart, permitting direct visualization of the cervix. Some manipulation may be needed if the cervix is far anterior or posterior. Once the cervix is defined within the tips of the speculum blades, the thumb screw is turned down to hold the blades separated. Note the presence and character of any

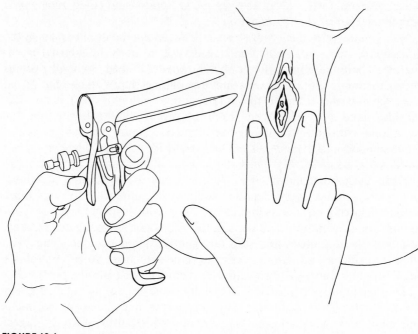

FIGURE 12-1
Introduction of vaginal speculum.

discharge. Is it thick or thin, watery or purulent, curdy or frothy, or malodorous? Does it appear to be vaginal in origin or is it coming from the cervix? Is the mucosa inflamed?

The next step is inspection of the cervix. Blood, mucus, or other debris may be swabbed away using small gauze squares or large cotton balls held in a long ring forceps.

Obtaining Specimens for Laboratory Examination

A sterile swab is used to obtain material from the cervical canal to culture for gonococci. These organisms are easily killed, so careful technique is important. Chocolate agar plates are used if the laboratory is nearby. Small bottles of transfer medium containing carbon dioxide are employed if the specimens must be sent to an off-premises laboratory. The culture medium should be at room temperature. This is best accomplished by setting a number of containers out of the refrigerator at the beginning of each half-day. If no suitably warm plate or bottle is available when it is needed, remove one from the refrigerator and warm it rapidly by holding it in your axilla for a few minutes. It is important not to turn a bottle of transfer medium upside down when it is open, because the carbon dioxide is heavier than air and would be lost if the container was inverted with the cap off.

Tests for diagnosis of herpesvirus and *Chlamydia* infections will also be indicated in some patients. The former can often be diagnosed by a Tzanck smear if suitable laboratory support is available, but viral culture is more often employed. Techniques for diagnosis of *Chlamydia* infections are in evolution and will not be discussed here.

Papanicolaou smears are obtained if this has not been done within an appropriate interval. Any mucus or other exudate should be removed with a swab before the cytological specimen is obtained. A sterile swab is inserted into the cervical canal, allowed to stay in position for a few seconds to absorb moisture, rotated gently to pick up some superficial cells, and withdrawn. Material from the swab is transferred to a glass slide using a rolling motion to minimize disturbance of cell architecture. The slide is sprayed with a preservative immediately to prevent distortion of the cells from uncontrolled drying. Products for this purpose are available from surgical supply houses; some brands of ordinary hair spray (Aqua-Net in particular) have been found to work just as well.

Use an extended-tip disposable spatula to obtain a second specimen for cytological examination. If the axis of the cervix more or less coincides with that of the vagina, insert the tip of the spatula into the endocervical canal and rotate it to obtain a scraping of superficial cells. If the axis of the cervix is perpendicular to that of the vagina, you may have to improvise a bit to obtain a suitable sample. This specimen, like the previous one, is spread on a slide and sprayed with a preservative. Keep your smears thin; they will not be readable if they are too thick.

If vaginal discharge or itching is present, obtain specimens for specific diagnosis. To examine for *Trichomonas* infestation, have your assistant place a drop of normal saline solution (no preservatives) on a glass slide. Use a sterile swab to obtain some exudate from the posterior fornix high in the vaginal vault, and mix some of it with the saline solution on the slide. Apply a coverslip. Examine the material under the microscope within thirty minutes. Preparations from patients with symptomatic *Trichomonas* infestations will usually show numerous motile trichomonads in a field with large numbers of pus cells. Trichomonads are slightly larger than pus cells and somewhat oval in shape with motile tail-like flagellae.

To check for candidiasis, have your assistant place a drop of 30% potassium hydroxide solution on a second glass slide. Pick a site with significant exudate on the vaginal wall, and obtain a vaginal specimen by scraping with a wooden paddle. Mix the two together on the slide. Apply a coverslip. Allow a few minutes for the potassium hydroxide to dissolve most of the cellular debris, and examine the specimen for *Candida* hyphae under the microscope. Many writers advocate the use of 10% potassium hydroxide solution rather than 30%, but if this is done, it may be necessary to heat the slide over a small flame to dissolve the cellular debris. Potassium hydroxide preparations are reliable if positive, but false negative results are common. Commercially available culture systems (Microstix Candida, Nickerson's medium) may be used to improve the diagnostic yield.

These tests are often helpful in the diagnosis of *Gardnerella* ("nonspecific") vaginitis as well. Normal saline preparations from patients with this infection may show "clue cells," epithelial cells which have a grainy appearance caused by the presence of clusters of bacteria on their surface. The potassium hydroxide preparation may also be useful in confirming a suspected *Gardnerella* infection. A characteristic "mousy" odor is given off when the specimen and the potassium hydroxide are mixed together (this is called the "whiff test").

Use coverslips on the slide preparations for these examinations both to protect the specimens from drying and to keep microscope lenses free of debris. If you neglect to use a coverslip or are careless in rotating the objective lens turret of the microscope, a portion of the specimen being examined may be transferred to the lens, rendering it opaque as the material dries.

Completing the Examination

After the necessary microscopic specimens have been obtained, turn the thumb screw of the speculum free. Remove it slowly, keeping gentle pressure on the thumb lever and inspecting the folds of mucosa for evidence of inflammation or tumors as they fall in place behind the blades of the speculum.

The bimanual examination follows. Start by palpating Bartholin's glands on either side of the labia and Skene's glands near the urethral orifice for masses or tenderness. Digital vaginal examination is usually done with the index and middle fingers together, although if the patient is virginal or if there is other reason to suspect that the opening will be small (for example, an older woman who has been sexually inactive for many years), it may be best to start with the index finger only. The opposite hand, applying gentle pressure over the suprapubic area, pushes the various organs down so that they may more easily be felt by the digit(s) in the vagina. Check the bladder; it should not be palpable unless it is full. Note the size, contour, location, and mobility of the uterus. Palpate in the area of the tubes and ovaries on either side of the uterus, noting any tenderness, sense of fullness, or discrete masses. If pelvic inflammation is suspected, move the cervix gently from side to side; when salpingitis is present, pain is frequently produced by moving the cervix toward the opposite side (chandelier sign).

Always keep in mind the characteristic physical signs of early pregnancy: Bluish discoloration and softening of the cervix (Chadwick's sign), softening of the isthmus between the cervix and the fundus (Hegar's sign), and enlargement of the uterus. Finding an adnexal mass with other evidence suggestive of pregnancy raises the possibility of ectopic pregnancy.

Sometimes it is difficult to reach high enough in the pelvis to accomplish an adequate digital examination. You may extend the range of your examination by indenting the perineum firmly but slowly with your examining hand. Tell the patient that you will be pushing fairly hard, and back off if the procedure causes discomfort.

Rectovaginal Examination

Changing the examining glove before rectal examination is recommended to eliminate the risk of carrying infection from vagina to rectum. It is of course essential to reglove if it is necessary to reenter the vagina for any reason after a rectal examination is done.

The final step in the pelvic examination is a rectovaginal examination, with the index finger in the vagina and the middle finger in the rectum. This procedure permits palpation of the cul-de-sac, rectovaginal septum, more posterior part of the pelvis, and distal rectum. If the uterine fundus is retroflexed, retroverted, or retrocessed, it may be palpable only on rectovaginal examination. Make an orderly assessment of all palpable structures, noting the size and position of the uterus and adnexal structures, and check for such anal abnormalities as masses and abnormal sphincter tone. If there is stool on the glove when it is withdrawn, test it for occult blood.

Special Aspects of the Pelvic Examination

The first pelvic examination.   A teenage girl's first pelvic examination is often a time of stress. She may suspect an unwanted pregnancy, be apprehensive that the physician or staff might disclose confidential information to a parent, or fear that the examination will be painful. There may be difficulty finding the right terms to describe her feelings and her sexual activities. She may be overly concerned that she will be thought to be ignorant, immoral, or both and therefore tend to overinterpret both the words and the nonverbal actions of her care givers, thinking that they are passing judgment on her. There may be a perception that she has little control over the doctor's actions or the events going on in her body. Failure to address these issues adequately may have adverse effects for the patient: She may be too apprehensive to give a complete and accurate history and too distracted to be able to absorb the advice you give her. She may become negativistic and refuse to follow your instructions. She may become so anxious that adequate examination becomes impossible and she avoids returning for further care. These considerations lead to the following precepts:

1. The physician and staff should be comfortable about their own feelings in dealing with sexual issues and should avoid being judgmental.

2. History taking should be done patiently, with care to avoid questions that imply certain answers, and in nontechnical terms appropriate to the patient's age and education. Take a few minutes to get to know the patient as a person, possibly inquiring about her school or work activities, recreational interests, and future aspirations.

3. The environment should permit complete privacy, and the patient should be assured that everything she says will be kept confidential.

4. If the patient is accompanied by a parent or other responsible adult, the initial history may be taken with that person present. However, the patient should have an opportunity to communicate with you in complete privacy. The physical examination should normally be done with only the patient, the physician, and (if a male physician) a female chaperone present.

5. The chaperone (nurse or aide) should play a major role in educating the patient, guiding her through the procedure, and simply being a caring person.

6. If pregnancy is a possible consideration, ask the patient before the examination how she would feel and what she would want to do if she is indeed pregnant. It's usually best to explore these options on a "what if" basis before the diagnosis is confirmed.

7. Try to give the patient some measure of control over the situation. Get at least tacit verbal permission to examine her. Assure her that you will do everything possible to minimize discomfort and that you want her to tell you if she has any pain during the procedure. Keep her informed of what you are doing at each step. Consider offering her the use of a hand mirror so she can watch the procedure and learn more about her anatomy.

8. Any lesions found should be explained in terms the patient can understand. Whenever possible, assure her that your findings are normal.

9. Perform the examination gently and without haste. Use a small, well-lubricated, warm speculum. Perform the digital examination with one finger first, and then introduce a second if it can be done without much discomfort. If vaginal examination proves too uncomfortable, you may be able to get the needed information with a bimanual rectal examination only, although some patients find the latter the most uncomfortable part of the procedure.

10. A complete pelvic examination can be performed in most adolescent patients if there is satisfactory relaxation. It may prove difficult, though, if the patient is anxious and tense. In extreme situations it may be wisest to do little more than touch the perineum, terminate the procedure, smile, and say something like, "Everything seems to be just fine, but I'll need to recheck you. Could you come back next week?" One should have to resort to examination under general anesthesia only rarely.

Examination during menstruation.   Routine pelvic examinations are ordinarily not performed during menstruation for aesthetic reasons and because satisfactory specimens cannot be obtained for microscopic examination. However, the presence of blood should not deter examination if it is clinically important, as for example in suspected miscarriage or appendicitis. A supply of menstrual pads and tampons should be kept on hand for patients who may have need of them.

The retained foreign body.   Occasionally a foreign body such as a forgotten menstrual tampon will be found high in the vaginal vault. Its presence can usually be suspected from the patient's report of an unusually foul smelling discharge. Remove the tampon during the bimanual examination, holding it between the index and middle fingers. As the object is withdrawn from the vagina, grasp the cuff of the glove with the opposite hand, inverting it over the fingers and tampon. When the glove is completely inverted, the tampon will be inside it. Tie a knot in the cuff to seal the object inside, and dispose of it.

CERVICAL PUNCH BIOPSY

Visible lesions on the cervix that might represent cancer should be biopsied. This can be done in the primary care setting if the services of a gynecologist are not readily available. Various types of biopsy punches are available for this purpose. No anesthesia is needed. The cervix should be cleaned well before the procedure but not in a way that traumatizes the lesion. Try to obtain your specimen at the junction of normal and abnormal tissue. Put it into a preservative (chosen on your pathologist's recommendation) immediately. If bleeding persists after the procedure and it cannot be controlled by direct pressure, apply Monsel's or aluminum chloride solution to the area or use silver nitrate sticks. It is sometimes helpful to alternate between applying Monsel's solution and silver nitrate until the bleeding stops.

ENDOMETRIAL SAMPLING

In primary care one most often wants to obtain endometrial tissue specimens to screen for cancer and premalignant endometrial hyperplasia, conditions that are most likely to appear in overweight, nulliparous women over age 50 with a history of late menopause. Material for microscopic examination can be acquired in various ways, none of which is free of drawbacks. "Vaginal pool" Papanicolaou slides are easy to make in the course of routine pelvic examination, but their false negative rate is about 60 percent. Scraping the endometrium with a small curette has a higher yield rate, but the cost is higher and there is still a risk of missing a malignancy. Complete dilatation and curettage (D and C) is the definitive diagnostic procedure, but its complexity is beyond the scope of this book.

The approach most widely used in ambulatory primary care is endometrial aspiration using the Isaacs or other type of disposable aspirator kits. The material obtained is spread on a glass slide and fixed and interpreted in the same way as a cervical Papanicolaou test. Like the endometrial biopsy this is a screening test not to be used for definitive diagnosis in the presence of abnormal bleeding or other signs suggestive of malignancy. Here is the procedure:

1. The contraindications of early pregnancy and endometritis are excluded by history and (if indicated) a pregnancy test.
2. A routine pelvic examination is performed, during which the axis of the uterine cavity is estimated.
3. Some authors advise cleaning the cervix with an antiseptic solution, while others consider this step unnecessary.
4. A tenaculum can be used to stabilize the cervix if insertion of the cannula is likely to be difficult.
5. Assemble the aspiration device in accordance with the manufacturer's directions. If using an Isaac sampler, slide the plastic sheath forward to the end of the cannula.
6. Insert the cannula gently the length of the uterine cavity, letting its tip pass through the plastic sheath as it is advanced.
7. Pull back on the syringe to create a suction, wait about three seconds, and release. Repeat this procedure two or three times,

moving the tip to a different area of the endometrial cavity each time. If a significant amount of fluid is obtained, detach the syringe from the cannula and discard the fluid.

8. Withdraw the cannula, eject material from its ports onto a glass slide using air pressure from the syringe, and fix the specimen in the usual way for cytological examination.

FITTING A DIAPHRAGM

A contraceptive diaphragm is a dome-shaped rubber device with a spring embedded in its rim. When properly placed in the vagina, it serves as a mechanical barrier to the migration of sperm from the vagina into the cervical canal. A diaphragm costs about as much as two months' supply of birth control pills and is essentially free of side effects except for an occasional case of contact dermatitis, a somewhat increased incidence of cystitis, and a small risk of toxic shock syndrome (TSS). Its effectiveness when used faithfully is less than that of the pill but matches or exceeds that of many other forms of contraception. Its limited popularity stems from personal and aesthetic considerations including the need to insert it before each episode of intercourse. Some women dislike diaphragms, but others find them highly acceptable. The ideal candidate for a diaphragm has a stable sexual relationship, is motivated to use the method faithfully, and is comfortable with the manual task of inserting and removing it.

Diaphragms are available in diameters of 60 to 90 mm in 5-mm increments. The size most often prescribed is 75 mm. The most common type has a simple coil spring in its rim. Diaphragms with more complex springs, usually the arcing spring or flat spring types, will fit better in some patients. Each user must be fitted individually and refitted after childbirth or any marked change in weight. Explaining the device and its use to patients is facilitated by plastic models (available from Ortho Company).

After routine pelvic examination, estimate the correct diaphragm size for the patient by feeling the approximate distance from the pubic symphysis to the posterior fornix with your examining hand. Determine the appropriate size more precisely by trial, using a set of fitting rings or trial diaphragms (Ortho, other sources). If the patient is tense during the fitting, the pelvic muscles may be tight; a diaphragm that fits properly at this time may be too loose later when the patient relaxes. Choose the largest size that will fit comfortably and have her return with the diaphragm in place to be rechecked a week or two later.

Diaphragms are slippery when lubricated and are tricky to hold when compressed for insertion. The technique of holding the device for insertion is demonstrated in figure 12-2. When a diaphragm is properly

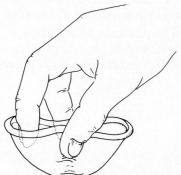

FIGURE 12-2
Method of holding diaphragm.

inserted, its posterior rim rests in the posterior fornix and the anterior lip fits snugly behind the pubic symphysis. The cervix can be felt through the midportion of the diaphragm. When the proper size is in place, the patient usually cannot feel it except by inserting a finger in the vagina. A few patients prove to be unsuitable candidates for diaphragm use because the anterior rim tends to lie at the introitus rather than anteriorly behind the symphysis. In others the cervix is so located that the diaphragm does not cover it. These problems can only be detected by a trial fitting. Have the patient remove the fitting ring or test diaphragm in your office. Recheck its position after she reinserts it.

Patient Education

Teaching a well-motivated patient to use a diaphragm is not difficult, but it takes time and must be done correctly if failures are to be avoided. The instructions should cover the following points:

1. Success with the method depends on using it properly and with every sexual encounter.
2. The patient will need to practice inserting and removing her springy, slippery diaphragm. This can be done in privacy at home.
3. A contraceptive cream or gel is applied to the rim of the diaphragm before insertion, and a dollop is placed on the surface that will lie against the cervix (it can be inserted with the dome up or down, as the individual prefers).
4. She should check to be sure that she can feel the cervix through the diaphragm ("It feels about as firm as the tip of your nose"). It's possible for the posterior lip of the diaphragm to catch on the cervix as it is being inserted. If this happens, the cervix will not be covered and there will be no contraceptive effect.
5. When the device is properly positioned, the patient is usually not

aware of its presence. If she can feel it (other than by digital examination), it probably is not in the correct position.

6. The diaphragm should remain in place a minimum of six hours and a maximum of twelve hours after intercourse.

7. To remove a diaphragm, the wearer inserts a fingertip between the diaphragm and the symphysis, catches the rim, and pulls it out. If this proves difficult, instruct her to do it in the squatting position while straining down (Valsalva's maneuver).

8. After the diaphragm is removed, it should be washed gently in mild soap and water, dried, inspected for pinholes against a bright light, and stored. The patient may dust some plain cornstarch on it, but talc and oily substances must be avoided.

9. Since the diaphragm usually is not felt when in position, it is possible for the patient to forget to remove it. This may lead to a malodorous discharge after a few days. The discharge usually resolves spontaneously after the device is removed. Instruct patients not to leave their diaphragms in unnecessarily because of the small but significant risk of toxic shock syndrome.

10. The patient may douche after removing the diaphragm if she wishes to, but it isn't necessary.

11. The patient may use the diaphragm to contain menstrual flow temporarily, as for example to improve the aesthetic acceptability of intercourse during menstruation. Because of the TSS risk, it should be removed promptly.

Ask the patient to return a week or two after the fitting with the diaphragm in place. This lets you reinforce your instructions and confirm that the device fits properly, and it gives the patient an opportunity to clarify any questions she may have about its use.

INTRAUTERINE CONTRACEPTIVE DEVICES

At the time of this writing most intrauterine contraceptive devices (IUDs) have been withdrawn from the market in the United States for reasons relating to the tort law system. They will be discussed here, however, in the expectation that that these devices, whose benefits exceed their risks for many women, will be available again in the future. The actual technique of insertion varies from brand to brand; the reader is referred to textbooks and the manufacturers' literature for details. The following general principles are pertinent:

1. As with all other forms of contraception, the patient needs to be

informed in advance of its advantages and disadvantages and to be an active participant in the choice of method. The adverse effects include infection, uterine perforation, impaired fertility, and heavy menstruation. Only selected aspects of the needed patient education are addressed here.

2. IUDs are usually inserted during a menstrual period, although the procedure can be done at any time if the possibility of pregnancy and pelvic infection have been excluded. The uterus is most relaxed during a menstrual period, and the risk of accidentally inserting an IUD into a pregnant uterus is minimized. It is also easiest to remove an IUD during menstruation.

3. Premedication is usually not necessary, but if desired a nonsteroidal anti-inflammatory drug may be given orally thirty to sixty minutes before the procedure. Under unusual circumstances one may elect to perform a paracervical anesthetic block.

4. Perform a routine pelvic examination, including determination of the uterine axis, before inserting an IUD.

5. Follow sterile procedure strictly. If possible, do not touch the IUD itself during the procedure, even though you are wearing sterile gloves. The cervix should be mechanically cleansed (not just swabbed) with an antiseptic, preferably an iodophor preparation.

6. A gentle approach will minimize discomfort and minimize the risk of perforating the uterus.

7. Accurate placement of the IUD within the uterine cavity is important. Follow the manufacturer's directions carefully with attention to determining the depth of the uterine cavity, and be sure that the IUD is placed in the transverse plane.

8. The monofilament strings used in many IUDs have a "memory" for shape and therefore may return to the contour they had in the manufacturer's package. Unless you leave the string long (usually about 3 inches showing through the cervix), it may curl completely into the uterus in time. If it cannot be seen or felt, you don't know whether it has fallen out or not, and sonographic or radiographic localization becomes necessary.

9. If radiography or sonography confirms that the IUD is still in the endometrial cavity, perform a pregnancy test before exploring for the string. The string can often be retrieved and the IUD removed using long, fine forceps or a spiral instrument made for the purpose.

10. Teach the patient to check for the presence of the string at the end of each menstrual period. If she cannot feel it, she should not rely on her IUD for contraceptive effect until its presence is verified.

SUGGESTED READING

Bertholf ME, Stafford MJ: An office laboratory panel to assess vaginal problems. *Am Fam Phys* 32(3):113, 1985.

Boone MI, Calvert JC, Gates HS: Uterine cancer screening by the family physician. *Am Fam Phys* 30(5):157-166, 1984.

Emans SJH, Goldstein CP: *Pediatric and Adolescent Gynecology.* Boston, Little, Brown, 1977.

Gelfand MM, Ferenczy A: Advances in diagnosis and treatment of endometrial hyperplasia and carcinoma. *Compr Ther* 9:12–23, 1983.

Hall DJ, Hurt WG: Lesions of the vulva. *J Fam Pract* 18:129–133, 1984.

Hamblin JE, Brock CD, Litchfield L, et al: Papanicolaou smear adequacy: Effect of different techniques in specific fertility states. *J Fam Pract* 20:257–260, 1985.

Hatcher RA, Guest F, Stewart F, et al: *Contraceptive Technology 1984–1985,* 12th ed. New York, Irvington Publishers, 1984.

chapter 13

Urological Procedures

CATHETERIZATION

Bladder catheterization in office practice may be done to obtain urine for laboratory examination from female patients who are unable to produce satisfactory "clean catch" specimens because of obesity, orthopedic problems, or vaginal bleeding or discharge; to change catheters in the ambulatory incontinent patient for whom other methods of control are unsatisfactory; and occasionally to check the residual urine volume of a patient whose bladder may not be emptying completely.

Catheterizing a patient with acute urinary retention in a primary care setting should be attempted only if a urologist or hospital emergency department is not quickly available and if the prospects for success seem good. A failed attempt at catheterization may increase the difficulty of subsequent instrumentation and can predispose to infection. Only practices located at a great distance from specialist services should stock the filiform catheters and other special instruments used by urologists for difficult catheterizations. In any case, do not remove more than 1000 ml of urine from the bladder at a time.

Catheterization may introduce infectious microorganisms into the bladder, especially if sterile technique is not followed carefully. Using excessive force in the procedure may cause the tip of the catheter to cut a false channel through the periurethral tissues. Paraphimosis may be caused by retracting the foreskin for catheterization and neglecting to replace it afterward. The procedure is uncomfortable, especially for male patients, although usually not enough so to require premedication. It is contraindicated if significant urethral injury is suspected.

Sterile disposable catheterization kits are available which contain gloves, drapes, germicide-detergent solution, cotton balls or swabs with plastic handles, water-soluble surgical lubricant, catheter, and a screw-top specimen bottle. A syringe and sterile water will be provided if a Foley catheter with retention balloon is to be used. A thumb forceps may also be included. An 18 French catheter is satisfactory for most purposes in adults; smaller sizes may be too flexible, tending to double over in the urethra if significant resistance is encountered. A smaller catheter with attached collection tube may be used to obtain urine specimens from women. Individually wrapped sterile straight and Foley catheters are also available, as are assembled complete closed systems including retention catheter, tubing, and collection bag. The chronic management of patients with retention catheters will not be discussed here except to note that the collection bag should never be lifted above the level of the bladder.

Procedure—Male

Patients are naturally apprehensive and perhaps embarrassed about being catheterized, so explain the procedure patiently and give assurance that you will be gentle. The patient lies supine, with an absorbent pad placed under his hips. A right-handed operator will usually prefer to stand on the patient's left. Open the kit with sterile technique, don gloves, and arrange the items for easy access. Apply the lubricant provided to the distal third of the catheter. Pour the prep solution into the bowl provided. If a Foley catheter is to be inserted, attach the filled syringe to the side tube and do a test injection to check the integrity of the balloon and tubing. Put a fenestrated drape over the penis, covering the surrounding skin. Grasp the shaft of the penis with your nondominant hand, and retract the foreskin if the patient is uncircumcised. Use your dominant hand to clean the glans and the distal half of the penis thoroughly, as your other hand holds its proximal half. Maintain sterility of the dominant hand by holding the prep swabs with a forceps or using swabs with plastic handles.

To straighten out the course of the urethra as much as practical, hold the shaft of the penis in a vertical position in men and in a horizontal (pointing toward the feet) position in boys. Hold the distal end of the catheter between the ring and little fingers of your dominant hand to keep it from swinging and possibly becoming contaminated. Grasp the catheter near its midpoint. Use thumb forceps if they have been provided, or else your thumb and index finger. As you continue to hold the penis upright with your nondominant hand, pass the catheter into the meatus and advance it gently. Resistance to advancement may be felt in the anterior urethra if there is a stricture, but in most patients the first resistance will be felt as the tip reaches the prostatic urethra and begins to curve cephalad. It will increase as the sphincter is reached. As the tip enters the bladder, resistance will decrease noticeably and urine will begin to flow. Let some run into a sterile basin, and then fill the specimen bottle. If the catheter is to be retained in place, advance it an additional 5 cm and fill its retention balloon. Most balloons hold 5 ml; catheters with 30-ml capacity are available for use after prostate surgery. Finish by taping the catheter to the abdominal wall or, if necessary, the thigh.

Procedure—Female

Catheterization of female patients is best done in the lithotomy position. The frog-leg position with a pillow under the hips may be used if necessary. The thumb and forefinger of the nondominant hand are used to spread the labia, in order to visualize the urethral orifice. Always swab the perineum from front to back to minimize the risk of fecal contamination. Identify the urethral orifice before picking up the catheter; slightly anomalous positions are not uncommon. Significant resistance to advancement of the catheter is seldom encountered once it has entered the orifice. The female urethra is of course much shorter than that of the male. In other respects the procedure is similar for patients of both genders.

SUPRAPUBIC BLADDER ASPIRATION

Obtaining uncontaminated urine specimens is sometimes important in evaluating infants with suspected sepsis or urinary tract infection. Suprapubic aspiration is simple to perform and carries low risk if done with careful attention to detail, but complications such as major bleeding and bowel perforation may occur. The test should be done when there is a significant volume of urine in the bladder, as demonstrated by ability to palpate the bladder and a dry diaper for at least one hour before the tap is done.

The infant is held gently but firmly in a frog-leg position, with one hand across the chest and the other holding the legs. The lower abdomen and upper thighs are cleaned well with a germicide-detergent preparation and cotton balls or sponges. A 22-gauge × 1- or 22-gauge × 1.5-inch needle attached to a disposable hypodermic syringe is introduced through the skin in the midline about 1 cm above the symphysis pubis. It is angled 10 or 20 degrees from the vertical, directed into the pelvic cavity. Maintain gentle traction on the plunger of the syringe, and stop advancing the needle when it is felt or seen to enter the bladder. Some authorities say one should stop if the first tap is unsuccessful; others would permit a second try with the needle at a 20- to 30-degree angle from the vertical. Since the needle tip may stimulate the bladder to contract, causing the infant to urinate, the procedure should be accomplished as rapidly as careful technique will permit. Apply a strip bandage to the puncture site when the tap has been completed.

Note: The technique of obtaining voided urine specimens is discussed in chapter 17, "Laboratory Procedures."

MANAGEMENT OF PARAPHIMOSIS

Paraphimosis is a condition in which the foreskin of an uncircumcised male subject, often a child, becomes fixed in the retracted position. The tight ring which corresponds to the orifice when the foreskin was in its normal position acts as a tourniquet, leading to swelling distal to the point of constriction. Sometimes the condition is caused by a physician or other professional who retracts the foreskin in the process of catheterization and forgets to replace it.

The first step in the treatment of paraphimosis is to grasp the penis with your stronger hand and gently squeeze out as much of the edema as possible. Gradually increase the force over perhaps a ten-minute interval. If this gives inadequate reduction, apply an "iced glove." Lubricate the skin of the penis from the contracted area to the glans with an anesthetic jelly such as lidocaine. Fill a large surgical glove partly with water and ice chips, and knot the cuff closed. Invaginate the thumb of the glove, and slide it over the previously lubricated penis. Leave it in position for ten or fifteen minutes.

Next try to reduce the deformity manually. Grasp the normal skin just proximal to the beginning of the edematous area between the index and middle fingers of your two hands. Place your thumbs on the glans, and apply steady pressure, attempting to pull the foreskin over the glans. Do not stop pulling until the foreskin has clearly come distal to the glans; one can be fooled on this point and stop too soon if the foreskin is still edematous.

If these procedures fail, a surgical approach will be required. Clean the penis well with a germicide-detergent preparation, and inject a local anesthetic without epinephrine along the dorsal aspect of the contracted ring. After draping and checking to be sure the area is anesthetized, make a longitudinal incision 1 to 2 cm in length through the tight area. It should be deep enough to allow the skin and subcutaneous tissues to separate but not so deep that the nerves, blood vessels, or corpora cavernosa may be damaged. Control any bleeding carefully, and close the incision transversely using running sutures of 4/0 gut or polyglycolate suture. If the incision was of adequate length, the contraction ring will have been relieved enough to permit reduction of the paraphimosis. However, the foreskin may now have a "beagle-eared" appearance, and the patient may choose to have a circumcision some weeks later after complete healing has occurred.

ZIPPER INJURIES OF THE PENIS

Boys and occasionally men can catch the skin of their penises in their trouser zippers. The resulting injury is painful, embarrassing, and sometimes frightening to the patient and family, but its prognosis is quite favorable. A few minutes for explanation and reassurance may pay major dividends in terms of decreased anxiety and enhanced cooperation. The top and bottom halves of the zipper slide are held together by the bridgelike piece at its upper end. It is a simple matter to use a compound-action wire cutter or surgical bone nipper to cut through this "median bar." When it is transected, the zipper teeth can be pulled apart, releasing the skin.

PENILE STRANGULATION FROM CIRCUMFERENTIAL OBJECTS

A variety of ring-shaped objects can be placed over a child's penis, and various types of thread can be wrapped around it, creating a tourniquet effect. In some cases the resulting edema will be so severe that the object cannot be removed except under general anesthesia. However, the offending object occasionally turns out to be a long piece of hair. This can be removed easily by soaking it for a few minutes with a commercial depilatory product (Nair, other brands) until the strands of hair dissolve.

VASECTOMY

Vasectomy, an operation in which the vas deferens is interrupted bilaterally, is frequently used as a method of male sterilization. It is normally done as an ambulatory procedure. Since negotiating with and educating the patient and spouse are as important as the technical aspects of the operation, vasectomy may be an ideal procedure for family physicians who will take the time to address all aspects of the procedure in a meticulous manner and perform it often enough to maintain technical proficiency.

Selection of Appropriate Patients

Start by deciding whether a permanent form of sterilization is appropriate for the patient or (preferably) couple who request it. Specific criteria vary; many would require either a stable marital relationship with two or more children or a mature (however defined) decision by the individual or couple that he or they will never in the future want to have children. Listen for inappropriate expectations, such as the couple where fear of pregnancy has been used as a reason for avoiding intercourse and the husband believes that removing this fear will improve their relationship. Be cautious also with those who think they will never want to be parents but are young enough that they may change their minds.

Some patients will have moral or religious beliefs that may make them reluctant to accept a sterilization procedure. It is the doctor's duty to help people clarify their values but not to impose his or her own.

Selection of Appropriate Sterilization Method

Vasectomy is a simple, relatively inexpensive procedure which carries little risk of serious complications and almost none of death. However, the male genitalia have such symbolic importance that many men are apprehensive about the operation. Physicians should explain its benign nature but should not attempt to coerce people who have mental reservations about its safety or possible effects on virility. Give the patient or couple the information they need, and let them choose among available alternatives which include sterilization of the woman and various reversible contraceptive methods.

Patient Education

Information about the procedure should be communicated to the patient and spouse verbally and in writing. For medicolegal reasons it is advisable to have two copies of a set of printed information at hand, one to be given to the couple and the other to be signed by them, acknowledging receipt of the information, and kept on file. The following topics should be covered:

1. Pertinent anatomy and reproductive physiology should be reviewed briefly, at a level the participants will understand. Note that the procedure only interrupts the flow of spermatozoa and does not affect the production and distribution through the blood stream of testosterone.

2. The procedure almost always causes permanent sterility (defined for the patient as inability to cause a pregnancy because of absence of sperm in the ejaculate). However, the procedure fails roughly once in four hundred times. Since failure is possible, it is essential that semen specimens be brought in at intervals after the operation to determine the absence of spermatozoa before other methods of contraception are discontinued. It usually takes ten to fifteen ejaculations after the operation before sperm are cleared from the tract. Other methods of contraception should not be discarded until two semen specimens, a month apart, have been found to be devoid of spermatozoa.

3. Late failures—six months or more after the procedure—are possible. Recommendations vary as to how long and how frequently semen examinations should continue, but checks at six and twelve months after vasectomy are not unreasonable.

4. The most practical method of producing semen specimens is masturbating into a clean container, either at home or in privacy at the physician's office. If the former option is chosen, the physician

should supply a suitable covered container which is not contaminated with soap residues or other possibly spermatocidal substances. The specimen should be brought to the office for examination within two hours. It should be kept close to body temperature, perhaps in the patient's axilla, in the meanwhile.

If the patient finds the above method objectionable, the best alternative is to have intercourse while wearing a special semen collection condom (Milex Products, Chicago) which contains no spermatocidal agents. However, sperm viability is not a major issue in this context: One simply wants to know if sperm are present or not. The patient should not have had intercourse for at least a day before the specimen is obtained.

5. Vasectomy should be chosen only as a permanent method. Reversal operations can be done, but they are major surgery and do not always restore normal fertility.

6. It is not possible to prove that vasectomy has no adverse health effects many years after the procedure is performed, but extensive research has shown no unequivocal evidence in this direction.

7. The patient should purchase a standard athletic supporter (scrotal support) and bring it in at the time of the operation; it will be worn constantly for two days afterward and longer if desired for comfort.

8. The procedure is done under local anesthesia. No sedation is required, although a mild tranquilizer can be taken beforehand if desired. A patient who has taken a sedative should not drive home after the operation.

9. The patient should rest quietly at home for two days after the operation to minimize discomfort and the risk of bleeding into the operative site. Applying an ice bag to the area for a few hours will reduce local swelling. Normal sedentary activities and intercourse can be resumed after two days, and other physical activities after one week.

10. Each skin incision will be closed with one or possibly two absorbable sutures which will dissolve by themselves in a few days. The patient should return for a follow-up visit about a week after the operation. If bleeding into the scrotum or major swelling of other causes should occur, a visit to the doctor should be scheduled promptly.

Preoperative Medical Evaluation

Ask the patient about any history of bleeding abnormalities, disorders of urinary or sexual function, or significant diseases of other organ systems which might be aggravated by an elective operation. Examine the genitalia and inguinal areas for anomalies, other diseases, and evidence of previous surgery. Check for minor skin infections which might predispose to wound infection. Laboratory tests are performed only if the history or physical examination raises questions that need further investigation.

The Operation

Many different techniques of performing vasectomy have been described, but that of Schmidt seems most practical and will be outlined here. The usual minor surgery tray contains most of the needed instruments; they should include an Allis clamp or towel clip to hold the vas during the procedure, some curved mosquito hemostats, and absorbable suture material such as 4/0 polyglycolate, preferably on a noncutting needle. There is also a need for a cautery device, either a small battery-powered one which can be sterilized or a sterilized needle electrocautery tip, the cord of which is connected to a small standard electrocautery machine.

Ask the patient to wash the area well during a bath or shower shortly before the procedure. Some authorities assert that the operative site should be shaved at home before the procedure, but this runs contrary to current knowledge of factors predisposing to infection. It is preferable to clip any hair that is likely to be troublesome with scissors, avoiding minor skin trauma which could predispose to infection.

Clean the scrotum, penis, and adjacent parts of the thighs and supra-pubic area well with an iodophor or chlorhexidine surgical scrub solution. Drape the area with sterile towels.

Grasp the spermatic cord gently between the thumb and forefinger of your nondominant hand, high on the scrotum at about the level of the root of the penis (figure 13-1). Inject the skin in this area with 1% lidocaine or other anesthetic agent, and then the underlying spermatic cord, aspirating frequently to prevent intravascular injection. Repeat this step on the opposite side.

Again grasping the cord and overlying skin, make a transverse skin incision about 1 cm in length, exposing the spermatic cord. Using a curved mosquito hemostat, dissect bluntly (by spreading the tips of the instrument) down to the vas deferens. The vas is readily identified as a firm, white, cordlike structure that does not bleed when cut.

Free the vas from its surrounding tissue for a length of 2 cm or so, and fix its position by passing a towel clip or Allis forceps around (not through) it. Transect the vas, and excise a short (5- to 10-mm) segment to be sent for microscopic examination. Sew a short piece of suture material to the specimen from one side for identification purposes.

Insert the cautery needle about 10 mm into the lumen of the abdominal

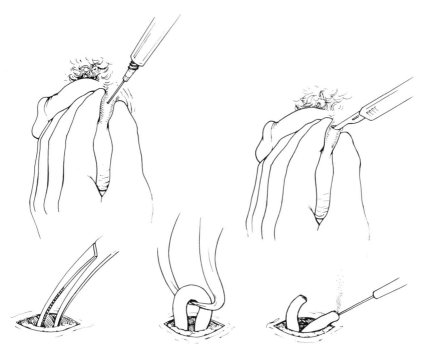

FIGURE 13-1
Technique of vasectomy.

end (farthest from the testis), and cauterize the lining and tip of this tissue conservatively. Then suture the surrounding connective tissue over the cauterized end to seal it off from the noncauterized end.

Check carefully for bleeding, and control any that is found with sutures or light cautery. Meticulous hemostasis is essential since blood diffuses easily through the loose connective tissue of the scrotum. Close the incision with one or (if necessary) two interrupted vertical mattress stitches of absorbable suture material. Use four knots, and cut the ends right at the knot. Repeat the procedure on the other side (figure 13-2).

A spray dressing such as Aeroplast or a wide piece of porous wound closure material such as Steri-strips may be applied. Have the patient don his scrotal support, with a sterile gauze square protecting the sutured incisions.

Two fine points should be kept in mind to maximize the chance of successful restorative surgery in the unlikely event that it should be attempted at some future time. The skin incisions should be made as high on the scrotum as practical so that the straight portion of vas is

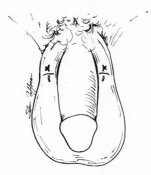

FIGURE 13-2
Completed bilateral vasectomy.

transected. Also, remove as small a pathological specimen as practical. Sending a segment of the vas to a pathologist for examination affords medicolegal protection but is not medically necessary since the crucial test is the disappearance of spermatozoa from the semen.

Aftercare

Instructions to the patient have been discussed previously, but some pertinent points will be repeated here. He should remain at rest at home for two days and avoid strenuous physical activity for a week. He should return if he observes major ecchymosis or abnormal swelling. He should bring a semen specimen in for examination after he has ejaculated perhaps twelve times; this will usually be enough to empty the tract of residual spermatozoa. He must not rely on the operation for contraceptive effect until two semen specimens (a month apart) have been examined and found free of spermatozoa.

One may, for medicolegal reasons, elect to have postoperative semen analysis done by an outside laboratory. However, formal analysis adds no useful information beyond what the physician can learn by simply looking at a fresh semen specimen under the microscope. You need only a yes-or-no answer as to whether sperm cells are present.

Complications

Vasovagal reactions may occur during the procedure, especially if there is traction on the spermatic cord. Reactions to the local anesthetic agent are occasionally seen.

Local swelling and mild degrees of ecchymosis are common after the procedure; they are treated with reassurance. Most hematomas are treated with bed rest and local ice; large ones must be evacuated in an operating room.

Sperm granulomas frequently appear in the form of small tender nodules in the tissues. Most can be left alone, but occasionally one must be excised for relief of pain. Recanalization of the vas seems to be more common in association with sperm granulomas, so extra semen examinations may be indicated when such lesions appear.

Superficial wound infections are occasionally seen; they are treated with appropriate oral antibiotics. Swelling of the epididymides may occur, but it is rarely bacterial and usually is treated expectantly.

Duplication or unilateral absence of the vas deferens may occur rarely. The former will cause a failed operation if it is not recognized.

SUGGESTED READING

Brownlee HJ, Tibbels CK: Vasectomy. *J Fam Pract* 16:379–384, 1983.

Pfenninger JL: Preparation for vasectomy. *Am Fam Physician* 30(4):177–184, 1984.

Pfenninger JL: Complications of vasectomy. *Am Fam Physician* 30(5):111–115, 1984.

Smith GL, Taylor GP, Smith KF: Comparative risks and costs of male and female sterilization. *Am J Pub Hlth* 75:370–374, 1985.

Weiss BD: Intractable urinary incontinence in geriatric patients. A management approach. *Postgrad Med* 73(4):115–119, 122–123, 1983.

chapter 14

Anus and Rectum

Consultant: JOHN W. DAVREN, M.D.

Most anorectal disorders can be managed in the family/primary care setting; skillful examination of more complex problems will facilitate accurate diagnosis and appropriate referrals. The ambulatory setting is also an appropriate place for the performance of flexible sigmoidoscopy, a powerful tool for the early detection of premalignant colon polyps and small bowel cancers.

EQUIPMENT AND SUPPLIES

Nonsterile, disposable plastic examining gloves are used, along with a water-soluble lubricant jelly (K-Y, other brands).

Disposable plastic anoscopes are suitable for most purposes (figure 14-1). Some physicians will prefer reusable anoscopes of the Hirschman type or perhaps those with a built-in light source (figure 14-2).

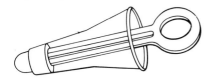

FIGURE 14-1
Disposable anoscope.

Equipment for sigmoidoscopy is discussed in the section on that procedure.

Disposable enema units, both saline and oil retention type (Fleet's, other brands), should be kept on hand.

If injection treatment of hemorrhoids is anticipated, the following items will be needed:

Long hypodermic needles designed for hemorrhoid injection, or 21-gauge spinal needles

Small syringes (3–6 ml) with finger rings to permit one-handed aspiration

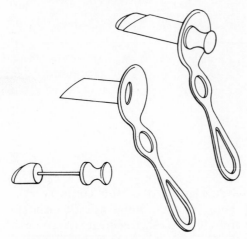

FIGURE 14-2
Hirschman anoscopes.

Sclerosing solution, 5% phenol in oil or 2.5% quinine-urea hydrochloride

If ligation treatment of hemorrhoids is anticipated, the following items will be needed:

Set of rubber band ligation instruments
Supply of special small rubber bands
Long Allis or similar surgical clamp

If treatment of thrombosed hemorrhoids and/or perianal abscess is anticipated, the following items will be needed:

Standard disposable 3-ml syringes with small needles
Ethyl chloride or fluorocarbon freezing spray
Surgical scalpel with #11 or #12 blades
Sterile surgical scissors
Allis or similar surgical clamp
Supply of sterile gauze pads

HISTORY AND PHYSICAL EXAMINATION

Since a good history often guides the physician to the performance of an examination that yields maximum information with minimum discomfort, careful questioning should precede the anorectal examination. What is the duration and time pattern of the symptoms? Has there been any bleeding? If so, is it fresh or clotted? Is it noticed on toilet paper, in the bowl, or on underclothing? If there is pain, does it appear only with defecation or straining or is it constant? Has there been anal intercourse, or have any objects been inserted into the rectum? Has the patient's life routine changed in any other respect recently (diet, physical exertion, psychosocial stresses)? Are there any systemic symptoms such as malaise, fever, weight loss, or change in bowel habits?

Explain the examination to the patient. Be sure he or she understands that it's normal to feel an urge to defecate during the procedure. Give assurance that you will proceed slowly and gently, and ask the patient to let you know if there is any significant discomfort. Simple digital examination and anoscopy of men is often performed with the patient standing bent forward with his elbows down on an examining table. Women are most commonly examined in the lithotomy position, usually in conjunction with vaginal examination. Either of the above positions may occasionally be appropriate in either sex. The left lateral decubitus (Sims') position is often the best choice for patients who are weak or acutely ill and is also preferred if a more extensive procedure is planned. The patient lies left side down with the long axis of the body at an angle to the table with the buttocks overhanging the side by a few inches (figure 14-3). Examination in the Sims' position is often made easier, especially in obese subjects, by asking the patient to lift the uppermost (right) buttock and hold it out of your way.

Inspect the perineum for evidence of dermatosis, excoriation, warts, fistulous openings, or other masses. Spread the perianal skin with a thumb on either side of the anus to look for a fissure, and ask the patient to bear down in an effort to demonstrate hemorrhoids.

Digital examination is performed slowly and deliberately with a gloved and well-lubricated index finger. Indent the perineum just anterior to the anus, and ask the patient to bear down. Allow a few seconds for the sphincter to relax as you ease the examining finger through the anal canal. Note the sphincter tone and the presence of any masses or significant tenderness. Search as high as possible for possible rectal tumors; with gentle but firm pressure you can indent the perianal tissues to permit the examining finger to reach a few centimeters higher. In men, note the contour, firmness, and degree of tenderness of the prostate gland. In patients complaining of pain near the rectum, check the coccyx and the muscles to either side of it. Pick up a bit of stool on your glove to be tested for occult blood, if possible. Hemorrhoids are usually too soft to be recognized on digital examination. Vaginal examination is discussed in

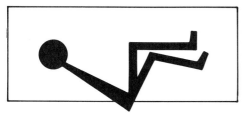

FIGURE 14-3
Sims' position.

chapter 12, "Female Reproductive Tract." Digital rectal examination is of course valuable in the diagnosis of many intraabdominal lesions, but these will not be discussed here.

Digital rectal examination can normally be performed with little difficulty in infants and small children if the patient and parent are reasonably relaxed. Use your little finger. The lithotomy position usually works best; it lets you watch the patient's face for signs of apprehension or pain as you do the procedure. Vaginal foreign bodies can sometimes be detected on rectal examination, and it may be possible to expel smooth objects by gentle digital pressure through the rectovaginal septum.

ANOSCOPY

Anoscopy is performed if there is a suspicion of hemorrhoids or other pathology inside the sphincter. Anoscopes come in many forms, but basically they consist of a cylindrical tube with attached handle through which the rectal mucosa can be inspected. There is an obturator to close off the end of the tube as it is inserted through the sphincter. Plastic disposable anoscopes are convenient to use and do not feel cold to the patient. Following completion of the digital examination, a suitable examining light is focused on the anal area, the anoscope (with obturator in place) is coated with water-soluble lubricant, and the patient is asked to bear down as the instrument is gently inserted to its full depth. The obturator is removed. Material for cultures may be obtained through the anoscope if indicated by the history or the appearance of the mucosa. The instrument is then withdrawn slowly as you examine the tissue falling into place behind it. Ask the patient to bear down once more to demonstrate the presence of hemorrhoids. Other lesions that may be seen include polyps, fistulous tracts, anal fissures, foreign bodies, and inflammatory processes.

Some anoscopes, such as the Hirschman type, have an angled inner orifice to permit better visualization of a portion of the mucosa. This is advantageous in the diagnosis and treatment of internal hemorrhoids, but two or three separate insertions must be made to do a complete examination with these instruments. Most disposable anoscopes lack this feature; they usually need to be inserted just once, but must be withdrawn more slowly and with greater care so that the entire mucosa is visualized.

SIGMOIDOSCOPY

Direct visualization of the distal end of the gastrointestinal tract facilitates the diagnosis of anal disorders, tumors, inflammatory bowel disease, diverticular disease, and other abnormalities. Examination of older patients at regular intervals is valuable as a screening procedure to detect early, asymptomatic carcinomas and premalignant polyps, thereby reducing morbidity and mortality from bowel cancer. However, no form of endoscopy short of total colonoscopy can be depended upon to detect all bowel lesions. There has been some controversy about the use of flexible sigmoidoscopes by practitioners without special qualifications in endoscopy, but many primary physicians have learned to use them well in structured continuing medical education programs designed to meet their educational needs. They start by practicing on plastic simulation devices before attempting the procedure, under supervision at first, on patients.

Two sizes are available: 35 cm and 60 or 65 cm. The former are less expensive and easier to master; the latter give more information. The use of colonoscopes, which are much longer and more difficult to use, should be reserved for those who obtain special training and maintain their skills by performing endoscopic examinations frequently.

The primary contraindications to sigmoidoscopy are conditions that might predispose to perforation, such as active inflammatory bowel disease or fixation of the colon from adhesions. Since flexible sigmoidoscopes are not completely sterilized between patients, it seems inadvisable to use them with patients who might be harboring dangerous pathogens such as the HIV virus; disposable rigid sigmoidoscopes may be used with such patients if the operator and assistants take other necessary precautions such as wearing plastic face shields.

Endoscopic biopsies carry significant risks, and in most settings primary physicians do not need to do them. Patients found to have bowel lesions will generally require referral to subspecialists who can obtain any needed biopsy specimens.

It's helpful to have an assistant present during the procedure to monitor and reassure the patient and to serve as "an extra pair of hands" for the operator. This person can advance the tube on verbal instruction as the physician sights through the lens system and manipulates the controls. Multiple-physician practices should consider the advantages of appointing one of their number to do all proctoscopic examinations for the group. Endoscopy, like most other manual skills, is done most rapidly, comfortably, and safely by those who perform it frequently.

Equipment and Supplies

Various types of instruments are available for such procedures. The traditional rigid sigmoidoscope is the shortest (usually 25 cm) and the least expensive to buy. It has been replaced by the newer types for most purposes, but may still be useful in settings where first cost is a major consideration. As previously noted, use of a disposable rigid scope may also be indicated in patients suspected of having infections that could be transmitted to patients subsequently examined with the same equipment. Use of flexible fiberoptic sigmoidoscopes requires more training and higher initial expense, but they yield much more information and cause significantly less patient discomfort. The flexible instruments are fragile and their glass optical fibers subject to breakage. Their life span is thus finite, but it can be prolonged greatly by gentle handling. Video endoscopes, which are coming on the market at the time of this writing, are even more expensive than fiberoptic instuments but promise greater image clarity, longer useful life, and a larger viewing image that can be shown directly to students, consultants, and the patient.

Retained mucus and small amounts of semiliquid stool are frequently encountered during endoscopy. A source of suction is needed for use with flexible sigmoidoscopes; this can be either an electric pump or an aspirator which screws onto a water faucet and operates on the Bernoulli principle. The former is more convenient, the latter less expensive. Long-handled swabs should be available to remove such debris during rigid sigmoidoscopy. Suction apparatus (pump, trap bottle, tubing, and a long metal suction tube) is optional but will make the job easier.

Preparation of the Patient

Informed consent for the procedure should be obtained, at least verbally, since there is a small but significant risk of complications. Sedative premedication is generally not required, but a short-acting benzodiazepine drug may be offered to selected patients. Antibiotic prophylaxis should be considered for patients at high risk for endocarditis or other complications of bacteremia. For most ambulatory patients a prepackaged phosphate enema, given an hour before the procedure, will provide adequate cleansing. Instruct the patient to hold the material as long as possible before expelling it; most people find it difficult to hold it much longer than ten minutes. Inappropriate enemas or the use of excessively harsh laxatives may cause irritation and spasm which interfere with the examination. You may wish to prescribe for bisacodyl (Dulcolax) tablets the evening prior to the procedure for some sedentary and/or laxative-dependent patients. An oral preparation called Golytely, taken in large volumes the evening before the procedure, is often recommended as preparation for colonoscopy. Enemas should be omitted in the presence of diarrhea or other evidence of inflammatory bowel disease.

Flexible Sigmoidoscopy

The 60- or 65-cm instrument and its use will be described in general terms. Use of the 35-cm instrument is similar except that the tip of some models can be manipulated in one plane only, and of course the depth of penetration is only about half as great. Become familiar with the particular brand of instrument you will be using and gain experience under supervision before attempting to perform the procedure on patients.

The *control head* contains the viewing lens, two concentric knobs which are used to move the tip in different planes, control buttons for air injection and suction, and inlet orifices for water injection and for passing flexible biopsy instruments down through the scope. The *flexible shaft,* containing the glass fiber optical system and other channels, is plastic-covered and has a metric scale to indicate depth of penetration. The tip, at the far end of the shaft, contains an objective lens and openings corresponding to those at the control head; its angle can be changed by manipulating the control knobs. A separate box, containing a bright light and a small air compressor, is attached to the instrument by a flexible cable which also contains a plastic hose for connection to an external suction pump. The instrument should be assembled and all phases of its operation (light source, suction, water and air insufflation, tip motion, and optical system) should be checked out before each use.

Explain the procedure to the patient, give reassurance that discomfort will be minimal, obtain informed consent, and verify compliance with your instructions for bowel preparation. Place the patient on a firm examining table in Sims' position: on his or her side, left side down, with the buttocks just over the edge of the table. The lower (left) hip joint is flexed about 90 degrees and the upper (right) hip about 120 degrees, with corresponding flexion of the knees. Portions of the patient that do not need to be exposed should be covered with a sheet. Wear disposable gloves. Inspect the perianal area, and do a digital rectal examination before inserting the scope.

Lubricate the distal portion of the shaft (but not the objective lens) with water-soluble surgical lubricant. Hold the head in your left hand, ready to manipulate the controls and to view the endoscopic image through the eye lens. Lay the tip of the instrument flat against the perianal skin with the right hand, pushing against it with the index finger to indent the skin. Rotate your hand, indenting finger and instrument together and easing the tip through the sphincter. Advance the instrument blindly but gently a few centimeters, stopping at the first sign of increased resistance. Insufflate a small amount of air to open up the lumen a bit, and advance the scope with your right hand under direct vision. Use suction to remove liquid debris from the bowel lumen. Inject water to wash off the objective lens if it becomes clouded.

The term "red-out" describes what one sees when the tip of the instrument is flat against the bowel mucosa. If excessive force is used the tissue blanches and one sees "white-out." In either case, withdraw the shaft a few centimeters, reorient the tip, and proceed. A small puff of air may help detach the mucosa from the tip of the instrument. Watch for abnormalities during insertion, but the most detailed and systematic inspection of the mucosa is done during gradual withdrawal. Always stop if the patient reports pain or if you can't see where you are going.

Keep the normal course of the bowel in mind. The axis of the anal canal is directed more or less toward the patient's umbilicus. There is then a turn posteriorly into the rectum, which generally follows the hollow contour of the sacrum. At a depth of about 15 cm one frequently encounters a sharp turn at the rectosigmoid junction, often anteriorly and to the patient's left. Ideally one should insert the instrument to its full depth, but this is sometimes prevented by inability to follow the sometimes tortuous course of the bowel, by spasm, by patient discomfort, or occasionally by the presence of an obstructing lesion.

Avoid aggressive advancement in the presence of inflammation or other lesions because of the risk of causing a perforation or other complication. Record the depth of maximum insertion.

Withdraw the instrument slowly, inspecting the mucosa systematically as you do so. Use the controls to look behind folds, "ironing them out" with the tip as necessary. Record the character, extent, and location of any lesions seen. As the tip approaches the rectum, aspirate excess air from the lumen for patient comfort. Finally, ask the patient to bear down to demonstrate the presence and extent of internal hemorrhoids as you withdraw it through the sphincter.

Rigid Sigmoidoscopy

The limited indications for this procedure have been mentioned previously.

The standard rigid sigmoidoscope is a 25-cm-long tube with a built-in lighting system. Its outer end is occluded by a glass lens whose point of focus is near the inner end. The lens is hinged so that it may be turned out of the way to permit removal of debris from the lumen of the bowel. There is a side nipple for attachment of a rubber tube leading to a hand-held inflating bulb. A removable rounded obturator is used to close the tube during insertion through the anal sphincter. Early sigmoidoscopes were made of metal; later models consist of a disposable plastic tube and obturator which are attached to a permanent lens and lighting system at the outer end.

One of three positions is used for the examination. In the *knee-chest position* the patient's weight is borne on the knees and shoulders. For stability the knees should be separated 12 to 15 inches. The abdomen hangs free and relaxed, "sagging like an old horse." The head is turned to one side for comfort. This position is uncomfortable, especially for weak or debilitated patients (figure 14-4). In *Sims' position* the patient lies on his or her left side with the legs flexed as described for flexible sigmoidoscopy. This position is easiest for the patient but (when using a rigid scope) most difficult for the examiner.

The two previous positions require only a plain examining table. The use of a *proctoscopic table* puts the patient in a position that is reasonably comfortable and affords ideal exposure from the physician's viewpoint. The patient kneels on a knee rest attachment and then lies down with the upper body supported on the shoulders, again allowing the abdomen to hang free. The table is then tilted perhaps 20 degrees into a head-down position (figure 14-5).

The initial steps of the procedure are essentially the same as described previously for flexible sigmoidoscopy: Enemas, explanation and reassurance, obtaining consent, and assembling and checking the instrument. Lubricate the exposed part of the obturator and the shaft of the scope. Wear gloves. Inspect the perianal area, and do a digital rectal examination. Then gently insert the tip of the scope (with the obturator in place) through the anal sphincter following the axis of the anal canal. Once through the sphincter, remove the obturator, close the lens over the end of the scope, and advance the instrument the rest of its length under direct vision. The anal sphincter becomes a fulcrum or pivot point for the advancing sigmoidoscope. To move its tip upward (toward the patient's back) you move the outer end downward (toward the patient's knees). Air inflation should be used sparingly to avoid cramping and distortion of the lumen. Debris may be removed either with suction or with long-handled swabs passed through the barrel of the scope.

Once through the sphincter, the tip is directed upward to follow the rectum as it courses through the hollow of the sacrum. At the level of the rectosigmoid junction, about 15 cm from the anal verge as measured by the scale on the shaft of the scope, one may encounter a sharp turn anteriorly and to the patient's left. It may be necessary to manipulate the instrument back and forth a centimeter at a time until the lumen beyond this point is visualized and the scope can be advanced farther. In some patients you will be unable to advance beyond the rectosigmoid junction because of sharp angulation of the bowel at that point. As with the flexible scope, most of the inspection is done while the instrument is being

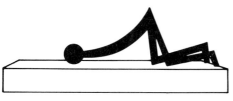

FIGURE 14-4
Knee-chest position.

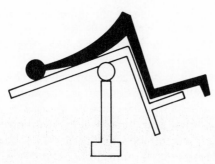

FIGURE 14-5
Proctoscopic table position.

withdrawn slowly from the highest point reached. A methodical spiral motion of the tip is recommended to ensure that the entire surface is inspected.

Cleaning

Scrupulous washing and disinfection of flexible sigmoidoscopes between uses is a matter of great importance for many reasons, not the least of which is the risk of passing infection from one patient to another. Personnel who do this work should wear disposable gloves and be careful not to splatter debris or contaminated solutions on themselves. The cleaning should be done promptly after the examination, before contaminants have had an opportunity to dry in place. The procedure includes washing the outside (but not the optical head), running cleaning solution and a flexible brush through the biopsy and suction channels, and exposing both the outside and the interior channels of the instrument to a disinfecting agent. Attempts at disinfection will be fruitless if debris has not been removed completely. Detailed instructions should be obtained from the instrument's manufacturer and followed carefully.

The tubes and obturators of disposable rigid sigmoidoscopes are discarded after use, but other parts of the instrument should be washed at intervals because they represent possible sources of contamination. Wash metal suction tips with soap and water, run soap solution and clear water through their lumens, and then autoclave them.

HEMORRHOIDS

Hemorrhoids are collections of blood vessels within the anal canal which may concern the patient when they bleed, ache, protrude, or facilitate fecal soiling. They are described as "internal" if they arise above the pectinate line, "external" if they arise below this landmark, and "protruding" if they are visible externally. In some patients the diagnosis is obvious on inspection; in others the lesions can only be seen endoscopically. Most hemorrhoids cause no symptoms and require no therapy. Some cause painless bleeding, although occasionally hemorrhoids represent a red herring in a patient who is bleeding from a more serious lesion higher up. Some hemorrhoids protrude through the sphincter and form tender masses, and a significant number develop painful thromboses (see following section).

Many forms of operative treatment have been advocated for symptomatic hemorrhoids. Those which are innocuous enough for office use (injection and rubber band ligation) are generally effective only in milder cases, while surgical hemorrhoidectomy is sufficiently painful that only patients with severe hemorrhoids will consider it beneficial. Cryotherapy is controversial; some writers find it useful but others consider the posttreatment inflammation and exudate too severe in relation to the benefits derived from the procedure. The mucosa below the pectinate line is exquisitely sensitive, while that above is insensitive to the usual painful stimuli (excluding traction and distention). Thus the relatively asymptomatic pure internal hemorrhoids can usually be treated without anesthesia, while the more symptomatic external and combined types cannot. A consideration of these factors leads to the recommendation that primary physicians should educate their patients on prevention and symptomatic management but should not undertake operative treatment of hemorrhoids, beyond managing acutely thrombosed external hemorrhoids, unless they have a special interest in the topic or practice in remote areas. Appropriate readings are listed at the end of this chapter.

THROMBOSED EXTERNAL HEMORRHOIDS

The patient with a thrombosed hemorrhoid, most often a young or middle-aged man, presents with a painful pea- to grape-size firm, violaceous mass of rapid onset at the anal verge. He may or may not have been aware of having hemorrhoids previously. There is often a history of recent unaccustomed physical activity.

Since the lesion is benign and self-limited, its treatment should be directed toward patient comfort. If it is relatively small and not very painful, one may prescribe nothing more than analgesics and rest, assuring the patient that symptomatic recovery can be anticipated in a week or two, although there may be a residual external skin tag. If the discomfort is more severe, the patient wants prompt relief, and the lesion has not been present for more than two or three days, immediate excision can be undertaken by the following method (figure 14-6):

The patient is placed in Sims' position with the affected side down and asked to pull the uppermost buttock out of the way to improve exposure. The mass and surrounding skin are washed, but no attempt is made to create absolute sterility. A local anesthetic such as lidocaine with epi-

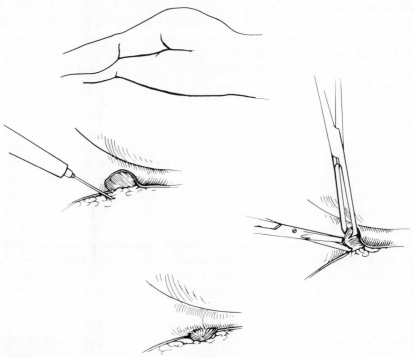

FIGURE 14-6
Excision of thrombosed hemorrhoid.

nephrine is injected into the skin and subcutaneous tissues at the base of the lesion. When satisfactory anesthesia has been achieved, the lesion is grasped with an Allis or other surgical clamp. It is then cut free from the underlying tissues with scissors, leaving an open defect about the size of a fingernail. No special aftercare is required beyond advising the patient to avoid straining at stool for a few days; the skin defect can be expected to close within ten to fourteen days.

RECTAL ABSCESSES

You may elect to drain a perianal abscess in your office if the patient is not toxic or in severe pain, if it is evident on rectal examination that the abscess does not extend above the sphincter and is localized in the skin and subcutaneous tissues about the anus, and if there is an obvious site for incision. The procedure can be accomplished as with abscesses elsewhere on the body (see chapter 3, "Nontraumatic Skin and Subcutaneous Lesions"). Patients who do not meet these conditions should be managed in a facility where adequate drainage can be done under general anesthesia.

FECAL IMPACTION

Impaction of stool occurs most often in physically inactive elderly patients. There may be a report of failure to defecate, or a paradoxical watery diarrhea may be present. The condition may also be picked up by finding a sausagelike left-lower-quadrant mass on abdominal examination. Digital rectal examination will reveal the presence of a massive, hard, usually lobulated fecal mass starting not far above the anal sphincter. Contraindications to removal are uncommon and include bowel perforation or risk of impending perforation, active inflammatory bowel disease, and other acute intraabdominal conditions.

To remove a fecal impaction, start by instilling perhaps 120 to 240 ml of mineral oil as an enema to be retained for an hour or two to soften the mass (disposable oil retention enema units are readily available commercially). Then, with old newspapers or other material on hand to catch the feces and a large plastic bag for disposal of the material, begin the process of digitally breaking up the impaction and extracting the pieces. On occasion it will be necessary to use other measures to stimulate peristalsis, such as a soapsuds enema, once the material within reach of the examining finger has been removed.

Be sure to address the cause of the problem in an effort to prevent a recurrence. This may involve dietary manipulations to soften the stools, attempts to increase the patient's physical activity, and judicious use of laxatives. Also, consider the possibility that the patient's failure to move his or her bowels is a signal that some unrecognized disease process such as an occult pneumonia is present.

SUGGESTED READING

Barone JE, Yee J, Nealon TF: Management of foreign bodies and trauma of the rectum. *Surg Gynecol Obstet* 156:453–457,1983.

Brenner BE, Simon RR: Anorectal emergencies. *Ann Emerg Med* 12:367, 1983.

Gordon PH: Management of anorectal abscesses and fistulous disease, in Kodner IJ, Fry RD, Roe JP (eds): *Colon, Rectal and Anal Surgery*. St. Louis, Mosby Company, 1985.

Frey KA: Rubber band ligation of hemorrhoids. *Amer Fam Phys* 29:187–189, 1984.

Katon RM, Keeffe EB, Melnyk CS: *Flexible Sigmoidoscopy*. Orlando, Fla., Grune & Stratton, 1985.

Lieberman DA: Common anorectal disorders. *Ann Intern Med* 101:837, 1984.

Weakley FL: Nonexcisional treatment of hemorrhoids, in Kodner IJ, Fry RD, Roe JP (eds): *Colon, Rectal and Anal Surgery*. St. Louis, Mosby, 1985.

chapter 15

Arms and Legs

Certain lesions which often appear on the extremities are discussed in other chapters. These include paronychias, embedded fishhooks, and the management of other embedded foreign bodies.

REMOVING RINGS FROM SWOLLEN FINGERS

Rings should usually be removed promptly from injured fingers. A ring may act as a tourniquet, aggravating any edema that appears subsequent to the injury. It may serve as a shield for pathogenic bacteria. Also, a ring may conceal a laceration that occurred when the finger was otherwise injured. In most cases the ring can be removed without difficulty. Sometimes the application of a lubricant such as soapsuds or surgical jelly will let it slide off. If the ring proves more resistant to removal, the "string method" will usually prove effective. Only rarely will it be necessary to cut a ring off. Ring removal should be accomplished promptly after the patient has been evaluated and the need for removal has become evident.

String Method

Bend a paper clip so that it forms a hairpin shape in one plane and a gentle curve in the other. Pass it under the ring, insert the end of the string in the loop, and pull it back so that the string passes under the ring (figure 15-1). Leave about 4 inches of string on the proximal side. Wrap the long end of the string around the finger, making a single spiral from the ring out to the base of the fingernail. The turns should not overlap, and there should be no gaps between them. Anchor the end temporarily by looping it under the preceding turn.

Now start uncoiling the string from the proximal end, pulling the short end at such an angle that the ring is gradually coaxed distally. As the string is pulled, the ring should pass slowly over the wide portion of the finger and then come free.

If the first attempt is unsuccessful, you can repeat the procedure. Stop pulling the string before the end slides under the ring. Pull it back to its

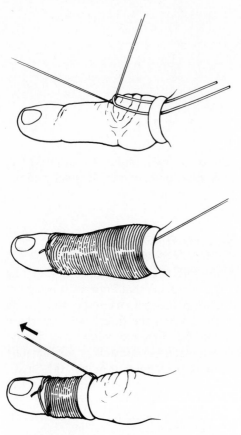

FIGURE 15-1
String method of removing rings.

original position, rewrap the finger, and try again. If this doesn't work, it will be necessary to use a ring cutter.

Ring Cutter

The ring cutter has two working parts which are approximated by forcepslike handles. One is a flat surface which is passed under the ring and serves as a protective anvil. Opposed to it is a cutting disk operated by a thumb lever. To use the ring cutter, lubricate the anvil and slide it under the ring. Then squeeze the handles gently to force the cutting disk against the ring, and rotate the thumb lever to cut through the ring. In most instances it will be possible to bend the ring enough to remove it after one cut has been made. If the ring is sturdy, it may be necessary to make two cuts on opposite sides of it.

Be sure not to lose the ring! Even if it has been cut, it is still valuable to the patient.

FINGER STRANGULATION CAUSED BY HAIR

Infants will occasionally wrap hair around their fingers or toes, causing acute strangulation and edema. Once swelling has occurred, it may be impossible to unwind the hair. This is an uncommon lesion but one where prompt, simple treatment can make a major difference in the outcome. Simply apply a commercial depilatory product such as Nair in the groove, work it in well, and wait for the hair to soften and break.

INGROWN TOENAILS

Ingrown toenails are a vexing problem which occurs most often during the second decade of life, involving almost exclusively the great toes. Their treatment has been considered to be difficult and unrewarding, largely (in the author's opinion) because of failure to consider physiological principles. A brief review of relevant anatomy and pathophysiology may help in understanding rational management. The nails are epithelial outgrowths which are formed by a matrix at their proximal ends. The nail migrates distally at a very slow rate. An ingrown toenail is one whose distal corner has curled downward enough to dig into the surrounding skin. It acts as a foreign body, causing an inflammatory reaction with edema, pain, and purulent drainage. A patient with a developing ingrown toenail often tries to cut the corner of the nail back diagonally to relieve discomfort. This process may be effective temporarily, but sometimes the person is unable to reach to the edge of the nail and a small hidden spur is left at its margin; this then digs in and stimulates an inflammatory response.

Many different forms of treatment have been advocated, varying widely in complexity and rationality. Soaking the foot and wedging cotton batting under the nail are sometimes recommended, although at best they give the patient something to do until the offending foreign body—the nail—is removed. Most writers advocate removing only part of the nail. Some advocate ablating part or all of the nail matrix. Some would excise a furrow along the lateral edge of the nail where it has lost support and tends to curl under. The literature is full of opinions and uncontrolled trials but little objective data.

In the author's view it is important to keep the procedure as noninvasive as possible. Since the circulation to the toes is not as abundant as that to other parts of the body, the risks of infection and delayed healing are higher here than elsewhere. The patients are usually young people who may be impatient with management programs that interfere with their normal activities and therefore unlikely to comply with restrictive treatment recommendations. The following approach seems as rational as any and has proven effective in practice:

The part of the nail which is acting as a foreign body should be removed at the first visit unless the patient is unwilling to give consent. In most cases the procedure should be done with a digital block, as described in chapter 2, "Surgical Principles and Technique." Once the block has taken effect, wash the toe with surgical soap. Take a sturdy pair of sharp-pointed scissors, and cut the nail in its long axis from the distal border back to the matrix, in such a way that about one-fourth of it, including the corner that is digging in, is cut free. With a strong needle holder or forceps, pry this piece of nail free from its bed and avulse it from the matrix. Any bleeding which may occur can be controlled with direct pressure. Dress the toe for a few days, using an antibiotic ointment to minimize odors and keep the dressing from sticking, until the skin closes over and drainage ceases. The use of systemic antibiotics is probably superfluous unless the patient is in some high-risk group.

There is difference of opinion as to whether one should destroy the matrix corresponding to the segment of nail that was removed. The author would not do so at the first procedure, but would if the problem recurs. Destruction can be accomplished in any of the following ways:

1. Use a small dermal curette to reach under the skin flap at the base of the nail, and curette the tissue in all aspects of this little cavity.
2. Apply liquid phenol to the same area to destroy the matrix, using a toothpick or wood applicator stick.
3. Do an *en bloc* excision of the matrix, using a suture or two to close the resulting defect.

Any of these procedures, if incomplete, may result in regrowth of a narrow spur of nail that must be excised later. The recent British literature suggests that this is least likely to occur with the application of phenol.

In some circumstances, especially if there is marked infection, it may be desirable to remove the nail by simple avulsion. This method carries a high incidence of recurrence but is simple and quick. Anesthetize the nail area with either a digital block or applying ethyl chloride spray until there is a frost on the nail. Take a sturdy hemostatic forceps, and force it under the nail, starting at the center of its free end and pressing the tip back to the matrix. Spread the tips of the instrument to separate the nail from its bed completely. Then use it to grasp the nail and pry it upward, avulsing it completely. With practice this procedure can be done in less than half a minute. Apply a bulky dressing, using an antibiotic ointment.

The patient should be taught to cut the nail straight across henceforth and let it grow long enough that its corner will be beyond the end of the skin and therefore unable to dig into the tissue.

SUBUNGUAL HEMATOMA

Crush injuries of the finger, such as those caused by a closing automobile door, frequently lead to hematoma formation under the fingernail. The same thing can happen if a heavy object is dropped on a toe. The lesion causes pain through pressure, and relieving the pressure relieves the pain. If the hematoma involves the nailbed, a new nail may grow out under the old one, gradually lifting it off its bed over a period of weeks to months.

Before opening the hematoma, check to be sure there is no associated laceration or fracture. The latter can often be established by grasping the distal segment of the finger from the sides and attempting gently to wiggle it laterally. If this maneuver causes no significant pain, the presence of a significant fracture is unlikely.

The blood is drained by drilling or burning a small hole in the nail over the hematoma. Hand-held drills, operated like a watchmaker's screwdriver, are cumbersome to use. Special electric drills are effective but unnecessarily expensive. Small disposable electric heating devices which have a small tip that becomes hot enough to burn a tiny hole in the nail are effective and easy to use. Lacking any of these, one can simply take a straightened paper clip, hold it with a hemostat, heat it with any available flame, and use it to burn a hole in the nail. It may be necessary to reheat the tip two or three times to finish the job.

Once the blood has drained out, apply a small strip bandage for a day or two to catch any residual drainage and reduce the risk of contamination. Further treatment is seldom needed.

RADIAL HEAD SUBLUXATION

In preschool children the radial head, which is not fully formed, may be pulled out of its annulus by a strong force along the long axis of the arm. This may occur if the child falls while being held by an adult or if the adult pulls on the arm in an attempt to control the child. The problem may be recurrent. There is discomfort in the arm which the child may or may not be able to localize. It is not severe as long as the extremity is at rest but gets worse with any activity. The child holds the arm in a position of slight elbow flexion with the hand pronated (palm turned downward). There may be mild tenderness at the site of the defect, but there is no redness or swelling. X-rays are normal unless there is an associated fracture.

The injury can be reduced easily without anesthesia or sedation. For an injury of the right elbow, use this procedure: Facing the child, hold the elbow in your right hand with your thumb over the radial head. Grasp the child's right hand with your left hand, and apply gentle traction to stretch the forearm between your hands. Then gently but firmly rotate the child's right hand into the supine (palm up) position. Relax the traction. There is usually a palpable popping sensation as the radius moves back into its normal position. Watch the child for ten minutes or so to see if he or she starts using the arm normally; this will occur in the great majority of cases. If it does not but you find no evidence for another injury, immobilize the arm with a posterior splint and sling and recheck it the next day. If normal function returns promptly, no further immobilization or treatment is needed.

SPRAINS

Sprains are tears of the ligaments which surround and limit the motion of joints. They occur when a joint is forced beyond its normal range of motion. In most cases the tear is partial, and the primary treatment is to immobilize the affected joint until the initial inflammatory reaction subsides and healing is under way. One then starts progressive mobilization to maintain the range of motion, muscle tone, and function. In more severe sprains there may be a risk of residual disability or increased susceptibility to reinjury; the management of such injuries is beyond the scope of this discussion.

Diagnosis

History taking should include the mechanism of injury, previous trauma to the same area, time interval from injury to treatment, and self-treatment before visiting the physician. It is important to know if the joint was temporarily dislocated but promptly reduced because this implies a major ligament tear. If the patient applied local heat to a fresh sprain, the doctor has a "teachable moment" in which to explain that heat can aggravate fresh injuries but that early cold applications will minimize edema and inflammation.

The *physical examination* involves palpation for areas of swelling and tenderness, gently testing for possible fractures, and checking range of motion. Identifying the specific ligaments that have been traumatized is relatively easy in the first few minutes after injury but becomes more difficult as edema and muscle spasm supervene. If the area is markedly swollen at the time of initial examination, it may be necessary to treat with ice, elevation, and compression and to defer definitive evaluation and treatment for a few days. Any false motion in the joint is significant, but one should not try too forcefully to elicit it. Be sure to check for other injuries which may have occurred at the same time and to note any coexisting muscular, vascular, or neurological impairment.

X-rays should be obtained in all but trivial sprains for medicolegal reasons and to pick up the occasional associated fracture which may not be evident on physical examination. Always examine the patient carefully before ordering x-rays; films should be ordered selectively depending on the precise location of the patient's injury.

Ankle Sprains

In most ankle sprains the mechanism of injury is forced inversion which stretches and tears the relatively weak ligaments of the lateral aspect of the ankle. Injury of the stronger deltoid ligament on the medial aspect is much less common. Examination begins with palpation to identify swollen or tender areas plus any clinically detectable fractures. After the possibility of fracture is excluded, one reproduces the mechanism manually to test for false motion. Attempting to move the foot forward in relation to the tibia and fibula (figure 15-2) may demonstrate rupture of the anterior talofibular ligament. Rotating the foot inward (figure 15-3) may elicit false motion of the talus in relation to the ankle mortise.

Ankle sprains are classified as first, second, or third degree. In first-degree sprains few fibers are torn, and prompt resolution without

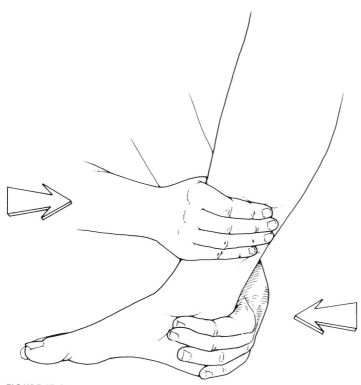

FIGURE 15-2
First test for false motion.

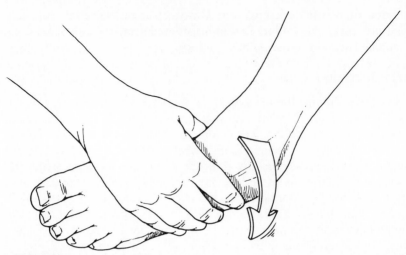

FIGURE 15-3
Second test for false motion.

residual disability is the usual outcome. Ice, elevation, and compression are the primary forms of treatment. Simple ankle strapping (see below) may give added comfort. In second-degree sprains more significant damage is done to the ligaments, and subcutaneous bleeding may be noted. More vigorous management in the form of a short leg cast has been advocated to minimize residual ligament laxness which may predispose to reinjury. Third-degree sprains are characterized by complete ligament disruption, false joint motion, and severe swelling and ecchymosis. There is difference of opinion on the relative value of prolonged immobilization and corrective surgery in these patients. Prompt orthopedic referral is indicated, since surgery will be most efficacious if performed within a week of injury.

The majority of cases seen in office practice can be managed effectively with adhesive tape and an elastic bandage. The purpose of taping is to restrict lateral movement involving the subtalar joint while permitting motion of the ankle joint itself in the sagittal plane. Many techniques have been advocated, but none seems better for most patients than simple "sugar tong" taping with an elastic overwrap. This is the technique:

1. Shaving or clipping the hair usually causes more problems than it solves, but it may be necessary for patients with unusually hairy legs.

2. Apply compound tincture of benzoin or other adherent agent in liquid or spray form to improve tape adhesion. Let it become tacky before applying the tape.

3. Sit on a stool in front of the patient who is seated on an examining

table (figure 15-4). Let the ball of the patient's foot rest on your knee. Hold the foot in midposition (90-degree flexion). Apply a single length of standard adhesive tape, 2 inches wide, firmly from just below the knee on one side of the calf under the heel to the same level on the opposite side. It is important that the tape pass under the heel, not the arch of the foot, so that it will not dig into the skin when plantar flexion occurs. This tape will usually stay in place for five days or more before it begins to work loose.

4. Apply an elastic bandage to the foot and ankle, with care to be sure it is not too tight. This minimizes soft tissue swelling about the injury

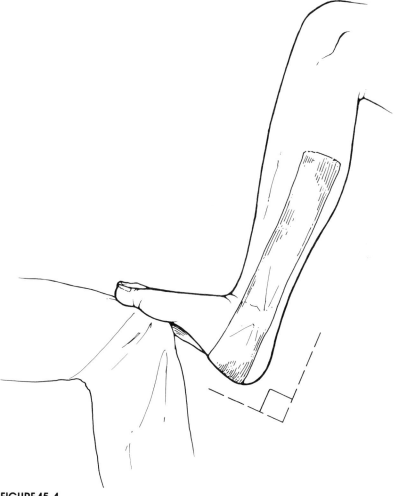

FIGURE 15-4
First step in ankle taping.

and also helps the tape to adhere to the skin (figure 15-5). The author favors a self-adherent elastic bandage (Coban, 3M Company), but if this is used, be careful to apply it less tightly than you would with other types of elastic bandages.

5. Crutches may be fitted if needed for comfort (see the section "Fitting Crutches"). The more soft tissue swelling there is, the greater the probability that weight bearing will be painful. However, cautious

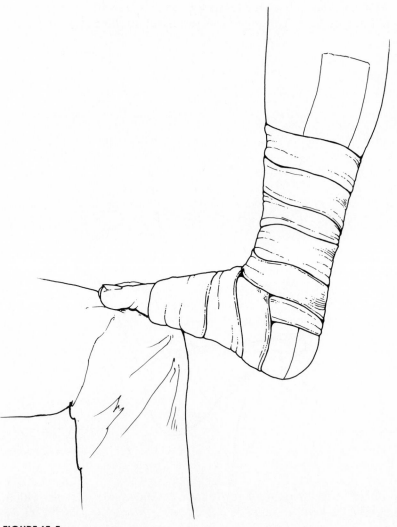

FIGURE 15-5
Completed ankle taping.

walking on a flat surface puts no significant stress on joint ligaments, so healing of an ankle sprain will not be retarded if the patient choses to bear weight on the affected leg.

Prescribe cold applications and elevation to minimize swelling. Analgesic–anti-inflammatory medicines may be employed as indicated. Use of the leg should be limited at first, with gradual return to full activities over perhaps a two week period, depending on the severity of the injury and the age and vitality of the patient. The adhesive strapping should stay on until it starts to come loose. The elastic bandage may come off when the edema is nearly gone. The patient can take showers without getting the dressing wet if a plastic bag is put on like a boot and held in place with a large rubber band.

Application of a posterior plaster splint and elastic bandage initially, followed by a short leg cast after the swelling has subsided, is currently favored for the treatment of ankle sprains in which there is a risk of residual ligament laxness after healing.

In some patients careful examination will reveal that the problem isn't in the ankle at all but rather at the base of the fifth metatarsal, where the peroneus brevis tendon may be avulsed from its insertion. Be careful in interpreting x-rays of this area; fractures do occur, but there is an epiphysis at the base of the fifth metatarsal which may persist into adulthood and lead the unsuspecting to diagnose a fracture erroneously. Avulsion injuries of the base of the fifth metatarsal are managed the same as mild ankle sprains.

Finger Sprains

The capsule of any finger joint may be torn as a result of being forced beyond its normal range of motion. If nothing more than an incomplete tear of the joint capsule occurs, the prognosis is favorable. So-called chip fractures, in which a tiny piece of the periarticular bone is avulsed along with the ligament, should be treated the same way as similar sprains without radiographic abnormalities (an important exception to this is the so-called mallet finger injury, described below). X-rays should be taken, but they cannot be relied upon to demonstrate more significant soft tissue injuries such as damage to tendons. The method of clinical examination for such trauma is beyond the scope of this discussion.

As with ankle sprains, immobilization for a few days is the primary mode of treatment. A variety of aluminum splints are available, either precut and shaped or in straight lengths ready to be cut to size with sturdy scissors. Plastic foam backing is often bonded to the metal for added comfort. It is important to shape any aluminum splint to the precise length and contour that will immobilize the affected joint in the position of function (figure 15-6). This will facilitate healing of the ligaments with maximal restoration of function and minimal residual laxness. Mild sprains of the interphalangeal joints can often be immobilized adequately with foam-backed aluminum "frog" splints (figure 15-7). They are held in place by friction and can be removed for hand washing, a major convenience. More severe injuries and those involving the metacarpophalangeal joints will need to be immobilized with aluminum splints which are long enough to reach to the base of the thenar or hypothenar eminence.

Mobility of the joint will decrease progressively if fixation is continued beyond one to two weeks. Gentle activity should be resumed promptly, under a formal therapy protocol if necessary. The time to full activity will vary with the severity of the injury and the age and lifestyle of the patient.

Important pitfalls in the care of sprains include the following:

1. One may focus on the sprain and miss an associated fracture or other significant injury.

2. The dressing used to immobilize the joint may be too tight (possibly causing local skin necrosis) or otherwise uncomfortable (leading the patient to remove it prematurely).

3. Progressive mobilization after the acute phase may be delayed too long, either through a lapse in guidance by the physician or from noncompliance by the patient. Reduced strength and mobility may result.

MALLET FINGER

If a blow along the axis of a finger forces the finger into sharp flexion, the extensor tendon may be avulsed from its attachment to the distal phalanx. This injury commonly occurs in failed attempts to catch a baseball. There

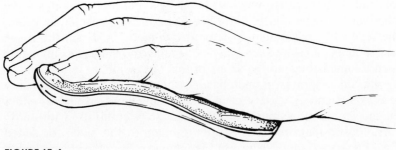

FIGURE 15-6
Application of finger splint.

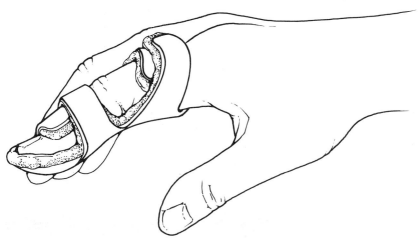

FIGURE 15-7
"Frog" splint.

may be an innocuous-looking "chip fracture" of the distal phalanx, but its presence is not necessary to make the diagnosis. The injury is diagnosed by demonstrating the patient's inability to extend the distal segment of the finger fully, although it can be passively extended by the examiner. Failure to recognize the injury and treat it promptly is often associated with a residual flexion deformity of the distal interphalangeal joint and inability to extend it fully.

The treatment of this injury is to keep the distal interphalangeal joint in a position of hyperextension until the injury heals, usually six to eight weeks. Proprietary splints are available for this purpose, or they can be improvised. They should contact all of the volar surface of the distal segment and almost all of that of the middle segment but should permit free motion of the proximal interphalangeal joint. During splint changes the finger should be pressed against a table or other flat surface to keep it constantly in hyperextension.

FITTING CRUTCHES

Since most patients for whom crutches are prescribed in primary care practices are not very familiar with their use, it is often necessary to spend a few minutes adjusting their size and instructing the patient in their use. The proper length is determined with the patient standing erect and with the tips of the crutches on the floor about 6 inches in front of and lateral to the patient's toes (figure 15-8). Adjust the total length to give two fingerbreadths of clearance between the top of the crutch and the patient's axilla. Then set the handpieces so that they are gripped

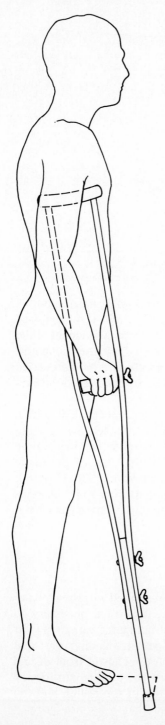

FIGURE 15-8
Fitting crutches.

comfortably with the elbows flexed about 20 degrees. Tighten the wing nuts after adjustment is completed, and instruct the patient to check them for looseness from time to time. The use of foam rubber pads on the handpieces may increase patient comfort and reduce the risk of blister formation during the first few days of use. Putting similar pads on the axillary crosspiece is less rational; the patient should not be bearing weight there anyhow, and the pads increase bulk which may predispose to brachial plexus compression.

Be sure the patient understands that weight is to be carried on the hands, not the axillae. Have the patient try out the crutches in your presence. Encourage development of a comfortable gait, swinging the legs through after each step. An occasional adolescent may need to be discouraged from trying to do too much too soon.

Teach the patient how to get into and out of a chair. When rising from the seated position, one holds both crutches in the hand opposite the side of the injured leg and braces the other hand on the chair's armrest. With an injured left leg, the right hand holds the crutches and the left hand is on the armrest. The same arrangement is used in sitting down; the patient should back up to the chair (on crutches) before starting to sit down.

SUGGESTED READING

Minor MAD, Minor SD: *Patient Care Skills.* Reston, Va., Reston Publishing Company, 1984.

Morkane AJ, Robertson RW, Inglis GS: Segmental phenolization of ingrowing toenails: A randomized controlled study. *Br J Surg* 71:526, 1984.

Roberts JR, Hedges JR: *Clinical Procedures in Emergency Medicine.* Philadelphia, W. B. Saunders, 1985.

Ruby LK: Common hand injuries in the athlete. *Orthop Clin N Amer* 11(4):819, 1980.

Saunders EA: Ligamentous injuries of the ankle. *Amer Fam Phys* 22(2):132, 1980.

chapter 16

Injections and Blood Sampling

STERILE TECHNIQUE: SOME REMINDERS

Sterile procedures applicable to primary care are straightforward and not difficult to learn, but a personal commitment to follow them faithfully is crucial if iatrogenic infections are to be avoided. Physicians should set the tone by following the rules themselves and by giving staff members the time, equipment, and support they need to perform all procedures correctly.

If a sterile object touches an unsterile one, it is no longer sterile and must be set aside. Lapses may occur if a needle tip touches clothing, hair, or unprepared skin or even if someone sneezes in its vicinity.

Skin cannot be rendered completely sterile, but its bacterial count can be reduced sharply by application of germicides *and* mechanical removal of bacteria and superficial contaminants. Neither is sufficient by itself. However, chemical or mechanical cleansing should not be harsh enough to damage the skin and impair its normal resistance to infection.

Almost all equipment for injection purposes is purchased prepackaged in sterile, disposable, ready-to-use form. Commercial sterile packaging is reliable only if it is protected from wetting and mechanical damage. Multiple-dose vials for drugs contain antimicrobial agents to reduce the risk that they will harbor and disseminate pathogens, but they must be discarded if it is known or suspected that contamination has occurred.

The techniques described below are considered procedures to be done by nurses or, in some cases, laboratory technicians. In offices without qualified personnel they may be performed by physicians. Some of them can be delegated to nonqualified personnel in some jurisdictions, but before doing so, one should investigate relevant rules and statutes and be sure the personnel involved are well trained and motivated.

Patients quite naturally do not enjoy being stuck with needles. Many little steps can be taken to minimize this discomfort:

1. Practice on oranges or other inanimate objects until you are comfortable with the technique. Patients are made more apprehensive

when they perceive that the person giving the injection lacks experience and confidence.

2. Complete the procedure as promptly as possible to minimize the patient's "worrying time." Prepare to do the procedure before you enter the patient's presence. If it may be necessary to restrain a small child, complete the necessary arrangements before the child learns what is going to happen.

3. Be honest, but not brutally so, about the pain you are going to inflict. Never say, "This won't hurt," especially to a child. Do, however, say something like, "I'll be as careful as I can" or "I'll get it over with as quickly as possible." Let the patient (and family, when relevant) know that you care.

4. Distract the patient with conversation. With youngsters especially, try to get the patient's mind on something else as quickly as possible after the procedure is done.

5. Let patients talk. Some will have factual questions that you can answer easily. Others simply want to say "I know you have to do this, but I don't like it." Still others may have deeper concerns about pain, risk of complications, or bad feelings that result from past personal or family experiences. Crying serves a useful psychological purpose and should not be discouraged.

6. Putting a small strip bandage over the injection site reduces the risk of soiling clothing and also serves as a "badge of honor" for children.

SUBCUTANEOUS AND INTRAMUSCULAR INJECTIONS

Subcutaneous injections are most commonly given through 25-gauge $\frac{5}{8}$-inch needles. Injection volumes are usually between 0.5 and 2.0 ml. The most commonly used site is the posterolateral aspect of the middle third of the upper arm. They can also be given over the anterolateral aspect of the thighs and the anterior abdominal wall.

Start by double-checking to be sure that you have the right patient, the right drug, and the right dosage. Expiration dates of all medications in stock should be checked monthly, but check again as part of preparation for an individual dose. If the drug is in a rubber-stoppered vial, clean the stopper well with an alcohol swab, invert the vial, inject a volume of air equal to the amount of liquid to be removed, and fill the syringe to the proper volume. If any bubbles form in the syringe, tap it gently so they rise to the base of the needle, inject them back into the vial, and withdraw liquid to the proper volume.

If the medicine is in a single-use glass ampule, it will be necessary to break the neck off the ampule. Most have a colored ring around their necks to indicate a weakened area that will break cleanly. Any that lack this feature should be scored with a small, disposable ampule file (usually supplied in the package). Tilt the opened ampule almost horizontal, holding it between the index and middle fingers of your nondominant hand, insert the needle into the ampule, and withdraw its contents into the syringe.

Clean the chosen injection site with an alcohol swab, and pinch the surrounding skin gently with your nondominant hand. Hold the syringe in your dominant hand as you would a pen, and insert the needle to its hub. Pull the plunger back to be sure the tip of the needle is not in a vein; if no blood appears in the syringe, push the plunger in to inject the drug. Apply pressure to the injection site with the swab as soon as the needle is withdrawn to minimize the likelihood of bleeding. Massage the site for a few seconds to encourage dissemination of the material through the tissues. Write the date, time, material injected, site, and your initials in the clinical record.

Intramuscular injections are given similarly, except for the site and the size of the needle. Larger volumes and more irritating preparations can be administered by this route. The traditional site in adults is the upper outer quadrant of the buttock. Recent writers have favored the ventrogluteal site on the lateral aspect, below the iliac crest but above the greater trochanter. It is important not to inject in the center or lower half of the buttock because of the risk of damaging the sciatic nerve. Small volumes can be injected into the lateral aspect of the deltoid muscle, with due caution to avoid the radial nerve. Intramuscular injections for infants and small children are given into the anterolateral aspect of the middle third of the thighs.

The needle diameter is a function largely of the viscosity of the material to be injected. Watery solutions can be given with 22-gauge needles; 19- or 20-gauge needles may be used for more viscous preparations. Lengths vary from 1 inch with children up to 1.5 inches for adults. Use longer needles for obese patients to prevent inadvertent and potentially troublesome injections into their subcutaneous fat.

INTRADERMAL INJECTIONS

The usual indication for intradermal injections is testing for immediate (IgE-mediated) or delayed (cell-mediated) allergy to inhalants, infectious agents, or drugs.

They are done with a short (intradermal) bevel $\frac{3}{8}$-inch 26-gauge needle and a 1-ml tuberculin syringe. The site most commonly used is the volar aspect of the forearm. The interscapular area is often chosen when multiple antigens are to be tested.

Clean the area to be injected with an alcohol swab, but not vigorously enough to cause irritation. Fill the syringe with the correct dose of the correct antigen, removing air bubbles completely. Grasp the forearm from beneath with your nondominant hand in a way that stretches the skin of the injection site. Hold the syringe between the thumb and fingers almost parallel to the patient's skin, with the needle's bevel upward. Advance the needle slowly into the upper layers of the epidermis until its beveled end is covered. Then inject the solution, raising a small wheal. Press the alcohol swab over the site of entry, and withdraw the needle. Do not massage the injection site.

Skin tests for immediate allergy are read after twenty minutes. Those for delayed hypersensitivity are read after two or three days. Measure the area of induration (not redness) with a millimeter scale.

ACCESS TO VEINS

In the primary care setting venipuncture is done to draw blood for testing, to administer medicines, and occasionally for fluid therapy. The sites used are almost always on the arms. The *antecubital area* contains the most prominent veins (assuming that they have not been damaged by multiple previous sticks) and is well suited to phlebotomy for laboratory tests. The *forearm* is well suited to infusions because the adjacent joints need not be immobilized. The *hands* are usually employed when other sites are inaccessible or have been destroyed. Veins in this area are superficial and easily seen, but they are relatively small and often tortuous. Access to veins on the backs of the hands is often made easier by resting the wrist and heel of the hand on a folded towel or other object, flexing the wrist joint.

Standard hypodermic needles may be used for intravenous injections. The shorter the bevel, the less likely they are to pass through the vein and out its posterior wall. Proprietary systems such as the Vacutainer simplify blood collection. Scalp vein administration sets are often useful on the back of the hand. Plastic cannula sets increase the comfort of intravenous infusions and reduce the risk of a needle coming out of the vein before the infusion is completed.

A tourniquet is applied to the upper arm to distend the veins for venipuncture. Various proprietary tourniquets are available; Penrose drain material and plain yellow rubber tubing are often used. If there is any question of the tourniquet being too tight, check the patient's pulse at the wrist. If finding a suitable vein proves difficult, try using a blood pressure cuff. Inflate it to a level no higher than the diastolic pressure. A common mistake is to allow insufficient time for the veins to fill before attempting to enter them with a needle. This may cause unnecessary pain for the patient and needless destruction of veins. Various procedures have been advocated to speed venous filling: Gently slapping the intended venipuncture site, having the patient alternately open and close a fist, etc. If access appears difficult, take plenty of time to search for the most promising site, looking on both arms, and then try to achieve access with a single stick.

In subjects with significant amounts of subcutaneous fat it is often possible to feel veins that you can't see. Learn to recognize the firm-but-yielding sensation of a distended healthy vein with your fingertips; it is quite different from that of a clotted or fibrotic vessel.

Once the site has been selected, clean it well with an alcohol swab. Hold the syringe or vacuum container system between the thumb and fingers of your dominant hand and begin the injection. Authorities differ as to whether the needle's bevel should be up or down; the latter position may be preferable if the vein is small and there is significant risk of inadvertently advancing the needle through the back side of the vessel wall. It is often helpful to stabilize the vein by flattening the overlying skin with the thumb and index finger of your nondominant hand or placing your thumb over the vein distal to the injection site. If the patient's subcutaneous tissue is lax and the veins move easily, look for a vein with a bifurcation, and enter it at the fork.

It is usually best to pass the needle tip through the skin with one motion and into the vein with a second one. The needle's entry into the vein is signaled both by a decrease in resistance to advancement and appearance of blood in the syringe. Release the tourniquet promptly unless continuing distention is needed to ensure adequate flow of blood for testing. When the purpose of the venipuncture has been accomplished, withdraw the needle and apply finger pressure for a minute or so through a small gauze square. Apply a strip or "spot" bandage.

LABORATORY BLOOD DRAWING

Blood is customarily drawn in clinical laboratories with the patient seated in a chair with a built-in armrest. Standard disposable syringes may be used, but a proprietary blood collection system such as the Vacutainer provides added speed and convenience. This type of system has three parts:

1. A plastic sleeve, open at one end and threaded at the other to receive the needle.

2. Special double-ended needles with a threaded collar at the middle.
3. Small test tubes with color-coded rubber stoppers. Air has been evacuated from them so that blood will flow in freely. They may or may not contain an anticoagulant, depending on the test(s) to be done.

Remove the double-ended needle from its container and thread it onto the plastic sleeve. Insert a tube in the other end until it impinges on the needle, but not far enough to break the vacuum. Clean the skin, apply a tourniquet, and enter a vein with the needle as previously described. Once in the vein, push the tube fully against the needle to let the blood enter it (be careful not to dislodge the needle tip from the vein as you do this). Release the tourniquet as soon as adequate blood flow is established. When the tube is full, hold a small gauze square over the entry site, withdraw the needle, and maintain pressure for a minute or so. Apply a strip or "spot" bandage. Remove the tube from the sleeve; if it contains an anticoagulant, rock it back and forth gently to mix the contents well.

To prevent backflow of contaminated blood from the vacuum container into the vein, have the arm tilted downward during phlebotomy, try to keep the blood in the tube from touching the stopper, and remove the needle promptly when the needed blood has been obtained. If multiple tubes are to be filled, use a needle with a sleeved inner needle. This will prevent blood flow while the tubes are being changed.

Note: The technique of capillary blood sampling is discussed in chapter 17, "Laboratory Procedures."

SUGGESTED READING

Fischer PM, Addison LA, Curtis P, et al: *The Office Laboratory.* Norwalk Conn., Appleton-Century-Crofts, 1983.

Nawrocki HR, West RS (eds): *Nursing Photobook: Giving Medications.* Horsham Pa., Intermed Communications, 1980.

chapter 17

Laboratory Procedures

Consultants: LUIS E. QUIROGA, M.D. and
ELMER F. WAHL, M.D.

Laboratory tests are essential to the accurate diagnosis of many medical problems, and they contribute to optimal continuing management of numerous chronic diseases. Doing these procedures "on site," when appropriate, speeds the decision-making process with benefits for both doctor and patient. The range of tests done varies widely among practices, and each practitioner or group must decide which to perform and which to send to an outside laboratory. The following are among the factors to be considered in making these decisions:

1. What level of expertise and interest in laboratory testing do your present physician(s) and other staff members have? Would it be beneficial to employ a laboratory technician or to arrange some training for the present staff?
2. Are you prepared to make the necessary commitment of time, funds, and supervision to ensure that your test results are always reliable?
3. What space and funding are available to start or upgrade the practice laboratory?
4. How easily can your patients utilize a commercial or hospital laboratory? Do you wish to utilize an outside laboratory through mail or courier service?
5. How much capital and operating expense for a laboratory can you justify considering the size, character, and financial resources of your patient population?
6. Are there any anticipated legislative or regulatory changes which might interfere with the function or financial viability of your operation? The laboratories of individual physicians and small medical groups are exempt from external regulation at the time of this writing, but that could change if widespread deficiencies in their operation become evident.

Quality control is a concern at all levels. Those performing the tests must be well trained and conscientious. They must have adequate physical facilities and supervisory support which encourages precision. Be sure that equipment is kept clean and maintained regularly and that supplies are stored properly and expiration dates honored. Specimens must be obtained properly, marked to prevent possible misidentification, and tested before deterioration can occur. Precise record keeping is essential. External quality checks, such as those available through the College of American Pathologists, should be employed. Duplicate specimens can be sent to outside laboratories for confirmation. Finally, results that seem clinically inappropriate (such as a negative pregnancy test in a patient with an enlarging uterus) and those with major implications for the patient's well-being (such as a white blood count suggestive of leukemia) must be confirmed.

Disease and injury in laboratory workers are not common, but they can occur if reasonable safety precautions are not followed. Do not permit pipettes to be filled by mouth suction because of the remote risk of sucking diseased blood or other specimens into the mouth. Needle sticks and glass cuts are avoided by care in handling and proper disposal of sharp objects. Food, beverages, and smoking should not be permitted in the laboratory. Purchase flammable substances in the smallest practical quantities, and keep them in secure and properly labeled containers. A large plastic squeeze bottle of an isotonic eye irrigating solution should be kept at hand for immediate use if any questionable substance splashes into someone's eye. Keep a dry-powder type fire extinguisher and perhaps a fire blanket close at hand, but not in a location where access to the equipment will be blocked if fire breaks out.

Interpret all test results with regard for their inherent variability and limits of accuracy. Space limitations preclude extensive discussion of this topic, but remember that most "reference values" or "normals" have been determined as statistical norms in limited populations and that slight variances—an urea nitrogen level of 24 or a white blood cell count of 4500, for example—do not necessarily signify disease. Be wary of technical errors too. Hematocrit determinations can be invalidated by inadequate centrifugation and serum potassium tests by conditions which permit hemolysis, for example. Do not hesitate to repeat and confirm abnormal results if in doubt.

The first test done in most office practices is dipstick urinalysis. The acquisition of a microscope permits more complete urinalysis, examination of vaginal specimens, and inspection of epithelial scrapings for fungi. Adding a centrifuge opens the way for hematocrits and microscopic examination of concentrated urine specimens. Inexpensive disposable tubes and pipettes are available for sedimentation rate tests. The purchase of a small countertop incubator permits cultures of the urine, throat, and vaginal secretions. Commercial kits are available for rapid diagnosis of pregnancy, streptococcal throat infections, and infectious mononucleosis. Finally, automated equipment may be purchased or leased to do blood chemistry tests and blood cell counts.

Some procedures will be described in specific terms in subsequent sections, but with many of them technology is advancing so rapidly that advice soon becomes outdated. However, manufacturers of new equipment have good reason to provide the instruction necessary to prepare their customers to use their equipment properly and will be very helpful if given the opportunity.

THE MICROSCOPE

The clinical microscope is a precise instrument of time-tested design which, if properly used and maintained, will give many decades of very satisfactory service. Selected parts and their use will be described starting at the base and working upward, since that is the direction in which the light travels.

1. A simple low-wattage light source in the base is sufficient for clinical use. A rheostat to control its brightness is a nicety, but a plain on-off switch will do. The light requires no attention beyond occasional cleaning and bulb replacement.

2. The condenser lens system, which focuses the light on the specimen, is moved up and down by a rack and pinion system. For most purposes it should be focused sharply on the grain of the light source's diffuser and then slightly defocused to provide light of uniform intensity. If you have trouble focusing the condenser lens, make an inconspicuous mark on the diffuser with a pencil and use it as a focusing target. For optimum image sharpness, refocus the condenser when switching from one magnification to another.

3. The adjustable diaphragm is built into the condenser unit. It is opened and closed by sliding a small metal tab. Close the diaphragm, and then open it just enough to provide adequate image brightness. Opening it farther will only degrade image sharpness by permitting scattering of light rays within the lens system.

4. The standard 1- by 3-inch glass slides on which smears and other specimens are mounted should always be used with coverslips, for many reasons. The most common problem when this rule is violated is that some of the material gets on the objective lens, dries in place, and severely degrades the optical image. Also, contaminants such as potassium hydroxide and urine can damage the objectives.

5. For most purposes one starts with the low-power (10×) objective, using the higher powers only when necessary to visualize small details. The 100× objective is always used with a drop of special immersion oil, forming an optical bond between the lens and cover slip. It is employed primarily to view bacteria and blood cells. Be careful not to get immersion oil on the 40× ("high dry") lens. Exposed ocular, objective, and condensing lens surfaces should be cleaned gently at intervals with high quality lens paper moistened with xylene, alcohol, or proprietary lens cleaning fluid. Other solvents could damage the cement which holds lens elements in place. The ocular and objective lenses may be removed occasionally and their inner surfaces cleaned with similarly moistened applicators. Let the surfaces dry before reassembling.

6. Get in the habit of adjusting the fine focus knob constantly while viewing a specimen. The depth of focus is often less than the thickness of the object; constant fine motion will help in perception of its vertical dimension.

7. Keep a dustcover over the microscope when it is not in use.

URINALYSIS

The primary indications for urine examination are screening during periodic physical examinations, diagnosis of suspected urinary tract infections and renal parenchymatous diseases, and frequent checking for protein and glucose in the course of prenatal care. Frequent urine examinations in diabetics are being superseded by home blood glucose monitoring. Urinalysis in the course of athletic physical examinations is controversial; most of the abnormalities found are innocuous, but detailed and expensive diagnostic evaluations may be needed to prove it.

Urine should be examined within a half hour after it is passed because cells and casts deteriorate, bacteria multiply, and odors form in standing urine. Specimens must be refrigerated if they cannot be tested promptly. A patient who is to bring a specimen from home should be instructed to wash the container well before filling it, even if it looks clean, because residues of powders or oily substances may appear as puzzling artifacts under the microscope. Sterile disposable specimen containers are stocked for urine specimens produced in the office. Less expensive unsterile containers may be used selectively when cultures are not likely to be indicated. The container should be marked for identification before it is given to the patient to be filled.

The more concentrated the urine, the more meaningful the examination. First morning specimens are desirable because they are usually collected after a few hours of water deprivation, but reasonably concentrated random samples are also reliable for most purposes.

Specimen Collection

Various procedures for obtaining clean voided samples have been advised, but complexity has not always been rewarded with better specimens. In presumably healthy men it is usually sufficient to provide a clean container and directions to the restroom. If a specimen for culture is desired, instruct the patient to start urinating into the toilet and then catch a "midstream" specimen in the container. If urethritis or prostatitis is suspected, give him two containers which have been numbered with a marking pen or grease pencil. Have him void the first few milliliters into the first container and the remainder into the second. Significant numbers of pus cells in only the first specimen suggest a disorder of the urethra or prostate, while their presence in similar numbers in both specimens indicates disease in the bladder or upper tract.

The situation is much more complicated in women for obvious anatomical reasons and for significant but less evident psychosocial ones. Women are more likely to acquire bladder infections than men, presumably because their urethras are much shorter. Voided urine flows somewhat irregularly over the labia majora, and the proximity of the urethral and vaginal orifices predisposes to contamination of urine specimens with vaginal and/or vulvar exudates. Some women find it difficult to follow explicit instructions for obtaining urine specimens.

Since vaginal contamination will make a specimen test worse than it should, not better, simple voided specimens may suffice for routine urinalysis in presumptively healthy women. If unexpected abnormality is found, especially if large numbers of epithelial cells are present, assume that vaginal contamination may have occurred and order a "clean-catch" specimen as described in the next paragraph.

If urinary tract infection (UTI) or other urinary disorder is suspected, instruct the patient on clean-catch technique or have it done by a well-coached nurse or aide (if the patient is obese or otherwise impaired, your staffer may have to assist her in the restroom). Swabbing the urethral orifice with antiseptic pads is often advised, but there is little evidence that it helps and povidone-iodine can give a false-positive reading for blood on urine dipsticks. The key steps in the clean-catch method are having the patient separate her labia, pass some urine into the toilet, "hold it" for a few seconds while the sterile container is positioned, and then void into it.

In some circumstances catheterization will be indicated, especially if a clean-catch specimen cannot be obtained. This is best done using a small disposable catheter or collection bag device. Proper sterile technique must be followed, both to obtain a meaningful specimen and to protect the patient from undue risk of iatrogenic infection.

Urine specimens can be obtained from infants by placing a sterile disposable self-adhesive specimen bag over the urethral orifice and waiting for the patient to fill it. If obtaining uncontaminated urine for culture is a matter of importance, suprapubic needle aspiration can be performed (see Fischer et al. in the "Suggested Reading" section).

Urine Examination

Urine examination includes some or all of the following steps, depending on the clinical situation:

1. **Gross Appearance.** Inspection of the specimen for color may suggest the presence of abnormal metabolites or of dyes such as phenazopyridine (these may interfere with dipstick testing). Turbidity may indicate infection, but it can also be caused by sediment such as amorphous phosphates; adding some acetic acid to a portion of the specimen will cause phosphates to go into solution, while turbidity due to infection will persist. Note any foul odor caused by urinary retention and infection.

2. **Concentration.** Measuring the concentration of solutes in a urine specimen is often neglected, but it is easily done and provides useful information. A dilute specimen may show falsely normal results on various test parameters. Inability to concentrate much above the isotonic level (sp gr 1.010, or 300 mOsm/L) may occur with renal diseases. Normal subjects should be able to concentrate urine at least to sp gr 1.018. The normal range, depending on water intake and other factors, runs from 1.001 to 1.030 or occasionally higher. *Visual inspection* of the urine obviously lacks precision, but very pale specimens are usually too dilute for reliable testing. The time-tested but much maligned *urinometer,* a weighted, graduated float which rides in a vertical glass cylinder filled with urine, gives data sufficiently precise for the needs of most ambulatory patients. Spin the float as it is inserted to discourage it from sticking to the side of the cylinder, and take the scale reading at the lowest point of the meniscus on the surface of the specimen. The *refractometer* permits greater precision but its cost limits it to high-volume laboratories. Multiple-test *dipsticks* have recently become available in which one segment gives an indication of the specific gravity.

3. **Dipstick Chemical Tests.** The modern multiparameter urine dipstick is a sophisticated disposable device which gives a remarkable amount of information at low dollar and time cost. The technology has advanced to the point where dipstick tests alone constitute adequate urinalysis in many patients. There are, however, many possible pitfalls in these procedures, and they should be considered only screening tests. Negative results may be accepted if consistent with the clinical picture. Abnormalities often require confirmation of one type or another. Manufacturers instructions must be followed with care to avoid erroneous results.

The tests available at the time of this writing include protein, glucose, ketones, blood, bilirubin, urobilinogen, pH, nitrite, leukocyte esterases, and specific gravity. The protein test is very sensitive, and trace amounts may appear in normal subjects. The glucose test is specific in that it does not measure other reducing substances. A positive nitrite test confirms the presence of gram negative bacteria, but a negative test is inconclusive. A wide variety of chemical and biological factors may occasionally interfere with these determinations; they should, as previously noted, be considered screening tests.

4. **Microscopic Examination.** New developments in dipstick tests, notable the leukocyte esterase procedure to detect granulocytes, have opened the way to an era of more selective use of urine microscopy. There probably is no need to do the latter on presumably healthy outpatients or those anticipating elective surgery if a full dipstick battery is normal. Microscopy may be avoidable in the ambulatory patient with dysuria who has no chemical abnormalities, although present evidence on this point is inconclusive. Patients with significant, unexplained organic disease, especially those who may have renal disease or lower urinary tract infection, deserve complete microscopic examination of the urine looking for cells, casts, crystals, and bacteria.

Some physicians prefer to examine uncentrifuged urine, but most authorities believe a more adequate examination can be done on centrifuged specimens. One simple approach is to centrifuge a tube of the urine (duration depending on the characteristice of the centrifuge), decant off about 95 percent of the supernatant fluid, add a drop of a stain formulated for this purpose (Sedi-stain, for example), mix the contents of the tube by tapping it briskly, transfer a drop to a slide with a disposable plastic pipette, apply a coverslip, and examine it under the microscope. Using the stain is optional, but it makes the various formed elements easier to see.

Examine the specimen for bacteria, leukocytes, erythrocytes, epithelial cells, motile trichomonads, casts, and crystals. The presence of large numbers of mature epithelial cells in a specimen voided by a female patient suggests the presence of vaginal secretions. If both epithelial cells and leukocytes are present in significant numbers, it may be necessary to examine another specimen, this time taking greater precautions against vaginal contamination.

5. **Culturing.** A number of proprietary urine culture systems are available for office use. Most permit presumptive identification of bacterial species and an approximate colony count. Some give information about antibiotic sensitivity. They can be useful in the management of uncomplicated urinary infections, although the more definitive capabilities of a clinical laboratory should be employed if the infection is complicated or if it does not respond to the initial course of antibiotics. In some instances it may be useful to take an incubating office culture to an outside laboratory for antibiotic sensitivity testing.

TOTAL WHITE BLOOD CELL COUNT

Note: Techniques for obtaining blood specimens are described in chapter 16, "Injections and Blood Sampling."

The total white blood cell count is widely used in primary care, most frequently in patients with respiratory infections as an adjunct to decisions about antibiotic treatment; in women with adnexal pain as an aid to the diagnosis of pelvic inflammatory disease; and in patients with abdominal pain to help identify those requiring surgical referral (appendicitis, cholecystitis, etc.). Less often it may aid in the diagnosis of hematological malignancies and various other infections.

Before automated cell-counting machines became available, white blood cells were counted visually under a microscope. Manual white cell counts are still useful in practices with limited capital resources and without quick access to an outside laboratory. The method is time-intensive and subject to technical error, but the equipment is inexpensive. The hemocytometer slide is a precisely machined glass object which is placed on the microscope stage for counting. It contains two flat surfaces on which fine grids, easily visible through the microscope, have been scribed. These grids define the area in which cells are to be counted. Adjacent to these surfaces are two slightly higher ridges. When the precisely flat coverslip supplied with the instrument is laid across these ridges, a chamber 0.1 mm in thickness is formed (figure 17-1).

Anticoagulant-treated venous blood is preferred for testing. Agitate the

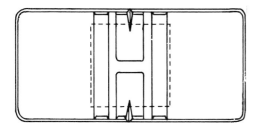

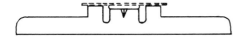

FIGURE 17-1
Hemocytometer.

tube before obtaining the sample to be sure it is mixed evenly. Finger-stick blood may be used if it is obtained with care. The blood should flow freely; wipe the first drop away gently and use the second drop for testing. Do not squeeze the finger. Finger-stick counts will be roughly 10 percent higher than those obtained with venous blood. The technique of diluting and counting white blood cells using disposable pipette-diluent units is described well by Fischer et al. (see "Suggested Readings") and in publications available from the Becton-Dickinson Company.

Automated blood cell-counting equipment has replaced manual counting in clinical laboratories. Significant capital outlays, technician expertise, and periodic maintenance are required, but precise results are available quickly at relatively little incremental cost. These instruments may be cost-effective in practices that do reasonably large test volumes and employ technicians familiar with their use. Their operation and care varies from brand to brand and will not be discussed here.

A new technology called *quantitative buffy coat analysis* has recently been described and introduced commercially. The principle of its operation can be understood by recalling that when blood is centrifuged in a tube, three layers appear: The red cells, being the heaviest, migrate to the bottom half of the tube. The plasma rises to the top. In between is a narrow light-colored layer called the buffy coat. It actually has three separable components: the granulocytic leukocytes, the lymphoctyes and monocytes, and the platelets. In the new system the length of the buffy coat layer is increased substantially by introducing a precisely made plastic float into the system which has a specific gravity intermediate between those of erythrocytes and plasma. It spreads the leukocytes and platelets out along the inner surface of the tube, making it possible to measure their volume, from which their number can be calculated. The parameters reported are hematocrit, granulocytes, lymphocytes and monocytes, and platelets. This technique involves substantial capital outlay but relatively little personnel time. It requires care and accuracy but is not complicated to perform. Initial reports of its accuracy have been favorable, but experience with the system is limited at this writing.

DIFFERENTIAL WHITE BLOOD CELL COUNT

Microscopic examination of stained smears of peripheral blood is a time-tested technique for estimating the relative numbers of different types of leukocytes and for determining the presence of abnormal cells of many types. It is labor-intensive and very dependent on technician skill but requires little capital investment. It is imprecise by nature, and the overlap between normal and abnormal values is often great.

Recent concern for cost-effectiveness in medical care has led to recommendations that the differential count be omitted from the standard "complete blood count" and be performed only when specifically ordered. The procedure seldom yields useful information when performed on asymptomatic patients. It may be helpful, though, in guiding further investigation of patients with undiagnosed physical illness. It sometimes aids in clarifying the significance of abnormally high or low total white cell counts and permits diagnosis of many erythrocyte abnormalities. It is reasonable, then, to obtain a differential count on "sick" patients, those with abnormal total white cell counts, and those with abnormal red cell parameters, but not as a screening procedure on people presumed to be healthy.

Like total white cell counts, differential counts may be performed on either venous or finger-stick blood samples. The same precautions apply to either technique. It is essential that the blood be smeared evenly and quickly on glass slides to prevent technical errors due to unequal distribution of different kinds of cells in different parts of the smear (figure 17-2). With experience one learns the size of drop needed to make a smear of suitable thickness which covers most but not all of the space available on the slide. Be sure to mark the slide for positive identification; this can be done with pencil on the frosted end of the slide.

The smear is allowed to air-dry and then stained with Wright's or a similar stain. Numerous modifications have been developed and are available commercially. One can either keep the staining solution in a special container large enough to hold a few slides at a time (Coplin jar) or else keep it in dropper bottles from which it is dropped onto slides as needed; the choice depends on personal preference and the volume of staining work done. Either procedure tends to be messy; suitable labora-

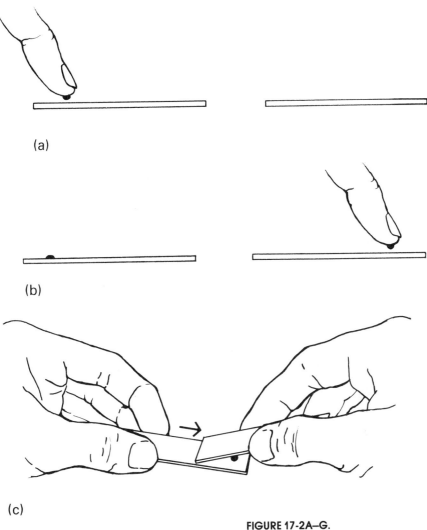

(a)

(b)

(c)

FIGURE 17-2A–G.
Preparation of blood smears.

tory space and staining trays will help contain the mess. Using forceps to hold the slides and wearing disposable plastic gloves will reduce staining of the operator's hands. Plastic aprons should be worn.

Immersion method. Stain the smear by immersing it in the solution for a number of seconds determined by the manufacturer's recommendations and trial-and-error experience. Then transfer it to a jar containing distilled water for a period approximating twice the staining time. Then remove it,

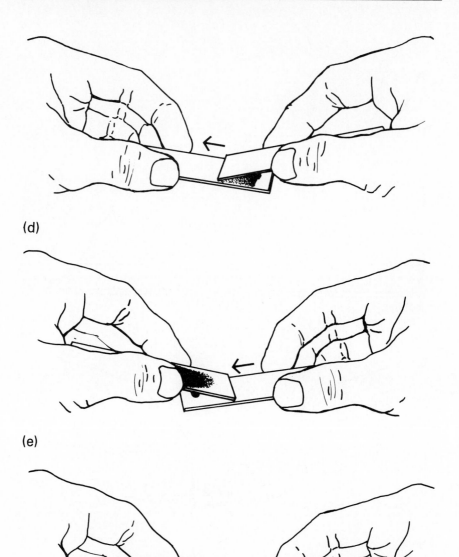

(d)

(e)

(f)

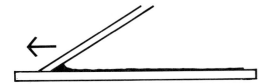

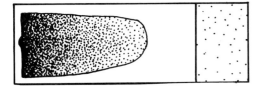

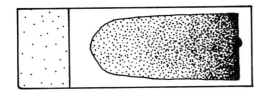

(g)

and rinse it by flooding it gently with water from a plastic wash bottle. Do not continue the washing process beyond the time needed to clear off the stain. Let the smear air-dry; do not attempt to blot it since it is only loosely adherent to the slide.

Dropper method. Place the slide in a completely horizontal position on a staining rack. Flood it with stain from the dropper bottle for a length of time determined by the manufacturer's recommendations and personal experience. Then apply an equal number of drops of distilled water, and mix the water and stain by blowing on them gently. Leave the mixture in place for an interval equal to twice the staining time, and then flood the slide with distilled water from a wash bottle to rinse off the stain. Let the stained smear air-dry.

Recognition and analysis of abnormalities in blood cells requires more training and expertise than most primary physicians are likely to have. Laboratory technicians are trained to recognize most hemocyte abnormalities, but those working in a primary care setting are unlikely to see enough of them to retain skill in their recognition. Hence the primary care office laboratory should concentrate on counting normal cells. Most abnormal smears should be referred to a consulting pathologist or hematologist. No attempt will be made to describe the many types of abnormal blood cells here.

MEASUREMENT OF ERYTHROCYTE PARAMETERS

Hemoglobin

There are few practices which cannot afford a Spencer hemoglobinometer (American Optical Company) or develop skill in its use. This instrument has been manufactured for decades and offers a simple, practical, economical, and reasonably accurate measure of hemoglobin levels. It is a hand-held instrument containing a light source, a colored glass wedge, and a small chamber for hemolyzed blood specimens. The chamber consists of two glass pieces, so arranged that there is a thin gap between them when the unit is assembled, and a metal clip and plastic handle which holds the parts together. The light can be powered by internal batteries or a plug-in power source. Hemolysis of specimens is obtained by use of small sticks impregnated with a suitable chemical.

Either finger-stick or venous blood may be used. Take the chamber unit apart and put a drop of blood on the shaped glass piece (with experience the proper size of drop will become apparent). Take a hemolysis stick, and move its coated end back and forth through the blood for a half minute or so until it becomes completely hemolyzed and clear. Apply the flat glass piece to complete the chamber, wipe off any excess liquid, and put on the metal clip. There are two sides to the chamber; be sure that the hemolyzed blood is in the side away from the handle. Insert the unit into the instrument. Press the button on the bottom of the instrument with your thumb to turn on the light, and move the slide back and forth until the light intensity appears equal in the two halves of the image seen through the viewing lens. Read the hemoglobin level opposite the mark on the slide. When the reading has been obtained, remove thumb pressure to let the light turn off and remove the chamber unit for cleaning. Simple water-washing and gentle drying are sufficient unless there is a buildup of residue on the glass.

There are additional scales on the side of the instrument graduated in percentages of various "normal" standards. These are archaic and should be ignored.

Many automated chemistry systems are also capable of measuring hemoglogin levels.

Hematocrit

The microhematocrit test is equally simple to do and is not much more expensive. It measures the percentage of the volume of whole blood that is occupied by red cell mass. It requires a centrifuge, either a small one made specifically for this test or one which can be adapted for the purpose. You also need a calibrated card for reading the results and a magnifying glass. Disposable heparinized capillary tubes and a puttylike sealant are the only supplies required.

The capillary tube is filled by touching it to a drop of finger-stick blood or a vial of venous blood. It should be filled approximately two-third full; a band on the tube provides a guide. Invert the filled tube, and press the clean end into the putty to seal it shut. Record the name of the patient and the number of the centrifuge slot into which the specimen was placed (running duplicate specimens is recommended). Centrifuge the specimen and read the result promptly. Lay the tube on the card absolutely parallel to the vertical lines, and slide it until the top of the supernatant plasma touches the 100 line and the top of the putty touches the horizontal 0 line. Read the hematocrit at the top of the red cell mass, ignoring the buffy coat.

Quantitative buffy coat analysis systems, described above in the "Total White Blood Cell Count" section, also provide hematocrit data.

Automated Hematological Testing

Red cell parameters can be measured with high degrees of accuracy and time efficiency on automated hematology testing equipment. Considerations relating to its use are discussed in the "White Blood Cell Count" section.

PROCEDURES FOR STREPTOCOCCAL THROAT INFECTIONS

Group A β-hemolytic streptococcal throat infections have been the subject of many studies and a significant amount of controversy through the years, partly because they represent a common upper respiratory infection which is responsive to antibiotic therapy and partly because there are late consequences of the disorder, most notably rheumatic fever, which can be prevented by accurate diagnosis and appropriate therapy. The situation has been complicated in the 1980s by the declining incidence of rheumatic fever, increasing understanding of the complex epidemiology of streptococcal throat infections, and the advent of simple diagnostic tests which can give a reasonably precise diagnosis in just a few minutes. There is presently no universally accepted standard of diagnosis; what follows is the author's recommendation based on personal experience, literature review, and attempts to predict the direction of future developments.

Clinical impressions as to whether a patient's throat infection is streptococcal or not are notoriously inaccurate. Throat cultures offer greater diagnostic precision than history and physical examination alone although there can be either false positive or false negative results. Their availability has improved diagnostic accuracy, both by giving reasonably reliable answers for individual patients and by informing physicians about the incidence of streptococcal pharyngitis in their communities at any given time. The most accurate culture methods require at least two days, which diminishes their usefulness in daily practice; surveys have revealed that practitioners often prescribe antibiotics while awaiting culture reports, which negates one of the claimed virtues of culturing, namely their potential for diminishing inappropriate use of antibiotics. The evidence currently available tends to support the view that antimicrobial therapy initiated in the first two or three days of the illness shortens its clinical course, but starting it later has only minor impact on symptoms.

The advent of rapid streptococcal testing promises a new era in which a precise diagnosis is possible before the patient leaves the office. The cost is somewhat higher than for cultures and false negative test results may occur; either or both of these considerations may disappear as the systems are perfected and economies of scale take effect. For the present a rapid test appears to be indicated for any child with a significant sore throat, any adult with pharyngitis and a history of rheumatic fever, and any adult whose symptoms suggest a high probability of streptococcal etiology. If the test is negative, consideration should be given to performing a throat culture as a backup procedure.

Many brands of rapid streptococcal diagnostic tests are available, each with its own advantages and methodology. No specific recommendations on technique or choice of brand will be given here because the field is evolving rapidly.

Many variations on throat culture technique have been advocated, but the following method is widely employed: Use a standard sterile disposable applicator to swab the posterior pharyngeal wall and/or tonsil to obtain a specimen for culture. The applicator should not touch the tongue, cheeks, or palate. Plate the specimen immediately onto a disposable sterile 5% sheep blood agar plate with the usual sterile precautions. Use a second sterile applicator or a bacteriologist's loop to dilute the inoculum by spreading it onto a fresh area of the plate. Flame-sterilize the loop, rotate the applicator 180 degrees, and dilute the material still further by spreading it into still another area of the plate (figure 17-3). Cover the plate, mark it for immediately with the date and patient identification, and put it in the incubator in the inverted position.

Examine the plate the next day, looking for small colonies surrounded by clear (beta) hemolysis. If any are found, select one or two that are distinct from other colonies; touch them with a sterilized bacteriologist's loop, pick, or a sterile wood applicator stick; and transfer each inoculum to a fresh sheep blood agar plate. Spread the inoculum well, and place a bacitracin disk on it with sterilized thumb forceps, pressing gently to be sure it is in solid contact with the agar.

Mark the plate for identification and incubate it overnight. Then read the plate for beta hemolysis which should be seen over the entire secondary inoculum except for a halo around the bacitracin disk. The ability of low concentrations of bacitracin to inhibit the growth of most strains of group A streptococci gives this procedure a relatively high degree of specificity.

Green (alpha) hemolysis on either the primary or the secondary plate may be ignored. If the primary plate shows no suspicious colonies when first read, incubate it for another day before calling it negative. No attempt is made to check antibiotic sensitivity in this procedure since the organism is almost universally sensitive to penicillin and erythromycin.

The agar plates are purchased from commercial suppliers. They are stored in the inverted position in a refrigerator until used. Discard any that become contaminated or outdated.

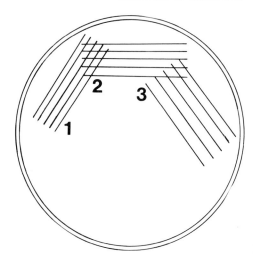

FIGURE 17-3
Method of inoculating agar plate.

If the bacitracin identification disk is applied to the original agar plate, a reasonably reliable answer to the presence of group A streptococci can be obtained in one day. This may be important in some clinical settings, although the advent of the rapid tests has diminished its significance. If the one-day technique is used, be sure the inoculum is spread out well and place the bacitracin disk at the junction of the second and third swabbings on the plate.

GRAM STAINED SMEARS

The Gram stain smear has many uses in primary care, including examination of urethral exudates for gonococci and defining sputum flora as a guide to therapy of community-acquired pneumonias. Urine specimens are sometimes stained to determine if significant numbers of bacteria are present; simple staining with gentian violet is often sufficient for this purpose. Specimens requiring other procedures such as acid fast stains should be sent to a clinical laboratory. Procedures for controlling the messiness inevitably associated with staining are discussed in the "Differential White Blood Cell Count" section.

A thin smear of the specimen to be tested is smeared on a standard glass slide and allowed to air-dry. It is then fixed by heating it over a flame (specimen side up); you can hold the slide at one end with your fingers, since glass is a poor conductor of heat. Heat the slide slowly until it is almost too hot to touch, and let it cool down before applying the stain. If practical, draw a circle around the specimen with a grease pencil to keep the stain from flowing where it is not wanted. Place the slide on a staining rack over a suitable tray or sink.

Different modifications of the Gram stain require different staining times; those specified here should be changed in light of personal experience and manufacturers' directions. Flood the slide with crystal violet solution for perhaps one minute, and then wash the stain off with tap water. Then flood the slide with Gram iodine solution for a similar interval, and again wash with tap water. Next tilt the slide, and wash it with decolorizing solution from a wash bottle until most of the color is gone; stop when the solution running off the slide no longer looks blue. Finally, flood the slide with safranine solution for ten seconds, rinse again with tap water, and let the slide air-dry. Slides which are to be preserved should be protected with coverslips, sealed in place with a drop of Permount or other protective sealant.

Gram-positive bacteria take up the crystal violet dye avidly and retain it through the decolorizing process; therefore they look blue under the microscope. Gram-negative organisms, on the other hand, lose the first color easily and appear red after being counterstained with safranine.

TZANCK SMEARS

The blisters of type 1 and type 2 herpesvirus infections and varicella-zoster infections often contain multinucleated giant cells. Demonstrating these cells under the microscope is a simple, rapid, and inexpensive way to confirm the clinical impression. The method does not differentiate among the different virus species.

Wear gloves to minimize the risk of acquiring the infection. Select an intact blister which does not appear traumatized or secondarily infected. Clean it gently and blot it dry. Unroof the blister with a scalpel blade. Blot out the blister fluid gently with sterile applicators or a cotton ball. Scrape the base of the blister with the scalpel blade to pick up some exudate, being careful not to cause bleeding. If bleeding occurs, start over with a different blister. Spread the scrapings onto a glass slide and let them air-dry. Apply one of the variants of the Wright stain (Hansel's or Giemsa's). One approach is to mix 0.5 ml of Giemsa's stain with an equal volume of tap water in a disposable hypodermic syringe, flood the slide with this mixture for thirty to forty seconds, and rinse it off. Let it dry, apply a coverslip, and examine for bizarre multinucleated giant cells, starting with the low-power lens and using higher powers as necessary.

SIMPLIFIED BLOOD GLUCOSE TESTS

The development of technically sophisticated but operationally simple methods of measuring the glucose levels of capillary blood samples has opened new horizons in the management of patients with diabetes. It has also simplified blood glucose testing in medical care facilities, including ambulatory care offices. Small practices which are not in a position to lease or purchase expensive, sophisticated, space-consuming laboratory equipment can do finger-stick glucose determinations with small, inexpensive, hand-held electronic meters. Test results can be available in just a few minutes.

Typically, a generous drop of blood is transferred from the patient's finger to a disposable single-use reagent strip, allowed to remain there for a carefully measured time interval, and then wiped off. A color change is read after a further incubation time, either in a special meter or visually by comparing the strip with a color chart. Most patients can learn to stick their own fingers, usually with the help of a small spring lancet system.

Patient education is important because of the risk that poor technique will lead to inaccurate results. Some manufacturers provide their own educational systems and will not sell their equipment without it. Some depend on medical office staffs to do the training. Others operate in the hope that patients will get the information on their own initiative. It is the physician's responsibility to determine that patients have received appropriate instruction and that their skills are monitored at intervals. This can be done by a knowledgeable member of the physician's staff if the patient volume is sufficient to justify doing so.

Most type 1 diabetics should be taught and equipped to monitor their own blood glucose levels. This is especially important for patients using insulin pumps, those whose control is unstable, and pregnant diabetics. The system may also be used as an adjunct to the care of selected type 2 diabetics. Difficulties may arise in patients who have poor vision, abnormal color vision (if a color chart is used), limited manual dexterity, or intellectual impairment. Checking the reagent strips visually against a color chart is somewhat less expensive than using a meter, but the test results are less precise.

In the medical office these systems can be used in screening for diabetes, following the progress of patients known to have the disease, and for rapid evaluation of patients suspected of having acute hypoglycemia. Recheck equivocal or unexpected results on more accurate equipment.

The technique is as follows:

1. The patient starts by washing his or her hands with soap and water. The site to be lanced may be cleaned further with a disposable alcohol pad, although this step is probably unnecessary. Either way the skin should be dry before the specimen is obtained.

2. A test strip is removed from the storage bottle and the cover replaced.

3. The spring lancet is loaded with a fresh disposable tip and cocked for use.

4. The patient holds the arm down at his or her side for a half minute to encourage blood pooling.

5. A site is chosen on the side of the distal segment of a finger and punctured with the lancet.

6. The finger is milked as much as needed to produce a large drop of blood.

7. The finger is turned over so that the blood is hanging dependent, and the drop is touched to the strip, being sure to cover the reagent pad(s) completely.

8. The contact time (typically sixty seconds) is measured carefully, and when it is completed, the drop of blood is removed. This is done in most systems by wiping with a cotton ball, although some require a water rinse.

9. After another measured interval (typically an additional sixty seconds), the result is read by comparing colors with a chart or by reading in a small meter.

AUTOMATED BLOOD CHEMISTRY TESTING SYSTEMS

Recent technological advances have made it possible for physicians and medical groups to purchase tabletop chemical analyzers which can perform complex biochemical tests with little need for technical skill on the part of the operator. Among the parameters that can be measured are glucose, creatinine, uric acid, urea nitrogen, bilirubin, AST, ALT, LDH, cholesterol, triglycerides, hemoglobin, sodium, potassium, and drug levels including barbiturate, phenytoin and theophylline. Others are in development. Supplies cost just a few dollars per test and the results are forthcoming quickly, but capital costs are significant. So many technologies and manufacturers are involved, and new developments in this field are coming so rapidly that only general principles can be stated here. Factors to be considered in leasing or buying automated equipment for in-office testing are discussed at the end of this chapter.

Instruction in use of the equipment is typically provided by the vendor. Periodic review of procedures is advisable. Do not set up for tests rarely done in your practice, both because supplies may tend to go out of date before they can be used and because one must do a procedure regularly to remain proficient in it.

EXAMINATIONS FOR PINWORMS

A presumption of pinworm (*Enterobius vermicularis*) infestation can often be established in an otherwise healthy child who complains of perianal itching, worst at night. The diagnosis is confirmed by visualization of the adult worms or ova. Pinworms live in the colon but migrate to the perianal skin at night to lay their eggs.

Sometimes parents can make the diagnosis with the "flashlight test." After the child has been asleep in a dark room for an hour or more, one gently spreads the buttocks and inspects the perianal area for threadlike off-white worms about one-half inch in length. More commonly, pinworm ova are harvested from the perianal skin and identified under the microscope. The highest yield is from specimens obtained at night by parents, although those obtained during office visits may be diagnostic.

Touch a disposable clear plastic tape with an adhesive surface to multiple areas of the skin around the patient's anus in an effort to pick up the ova. This can be done with disposable specimen collectors made for the purpose, or one can attach a piece of ordinary cellophane tape to a tongue blade with a portion of the stick surface exposed (figure 17-4). Put a drop of toluene or xylene on a microscope slide, and affix the tape over it, sticky side down. Examine the specimen under low power and reduced light, looking for double-walled ova which are flat on one side and roughly the size of an epithelial cell.

EXAMINATION FOR NASAL EOSINOPHILIA

Examining nasal secretions for eosinophils is a simple but useful adjunct in the diagnosis of allergic rhinitis. The patient is asked to blow his or her nose into a piece of household waxed paper. Some of the material is smeared onto a glass slide with an ordinary cotton-tipped applicator and permitted to air-dry. It is then stained with Wright's stain or one of its modifications.

After staining is completed and the slide has dried, it is scanned in a systematic manner under the oil immersion lens. The leukocytes are inspected, and an estimate of the proportion that are eosinophilic is made. Four percent eosinophils or more is considered diagnostic of allergic rhinitis. The test is reasonably reliable if positive, but not absolutely diagnostic.

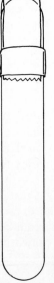

FIGURE 17-4
Device for harvesting pinworms.

ADDITIONAL TESTS WORTH PERFORMING

Only general statements can be given here with regard to some useful tests because of rapid technological advancements, frequent modifications of established tests, and the need to follow manufacturers' directions carefully. However, the following are appropriate procedures for many primary care practices:

1. **Tests for Occult Blood in the Stool.** The rationale for these tests is simple enough: Gastrointestinal malignancies and premalignant lesions may shed small amounts of blood into the bowel, and detecting this blood may trigger life-saving diagnostic studies. The sensitivity level of currently available procedures is high enough to detect most pathological bleeding and low enough to minimize detection of insignificant amounts of blood. The tests are inexpensive, simple to perform, and give immediate results. There are drawbacks, though. Cancers often bleed intermittently, and single or even multiple tests may be falsely negative. Numerous foods and other substances can interfere with the results, in either direction.

   Some physicians are more strict than others about instructing patients on avoidance of meat, vitamin C, and vegetables with peroxidase activity prior to obtaining specimens for testing. If these procedures are not followed and a positive result is obtained, consider repeating them after three days on restricted intake before ordering more expensive and invasive testing.

   Although the evidence that stool tests for occult blood can save lives is far from conclusive, they can be recommended as screening procedures at the time of routine physical examinations, probably starting at age 40. Older patients should be advised to obtain multiple specimens at home at intervals, checking three separate bowel movements and returning the slides to the medical facility to be developed and read. The procedure is also useful in many other clinical situations where occult intestinal bleeding is suspected.

2. **Pregnancy Tests.** A prompt, reliable answer as to whether a patient is pregnant or not is often a matter of personal significance to the family involved and occasionally (if elective abortion is contemplated or ectopic pregnancy is suspected) of great importance. The available tests vary in sensitivity, complexity, reliability, and cost. Serum tests are generally more sensitive and more expensive than urine tests, and tube tests are often more sensitive than slide tests. Urine specimens with a specific gravity of less than 1.010 are unreliable; concentrated first morning specimens are preferred.

3. **Tests for Infectious Mononucleosis.** Slide tests for infectious mononucleosis are reasonably accurate. They may not become positive

until the patient has had symptoms for a week or more.

Note: The examination of vaginal secretions is addressed in chapter 12, "Female Reproductive Tract."

PREPARATION OF TEACHING SLIDES

Properly stained and washed hematological and Gram stain smears will remain usable for many years if a coverslip is applied and secured with an adhesive-preservative preparation such as Permount or Pro-Texx. Parasitic ova and pinworms can be preserved in the same way. Liquid preparations such as stained urine specimens will sometimes remain readable for some weeks if the edges of the coverslip are sealed with the same product. Their life can be prolonged by adding a small amount of glutaraldehyde 2% solution to the specimen. Slides should be stored in a dark place to minimize deterioration of dyes.

Physicians with an interest in photography who have access to a 35-mm interchangeable-lens single-reflex camera can learn to make high-quality photographic slides through a microscope. The only equipment purchases required are a microscope adapter and a right-angle viewfinder to fit the particular brand of camera on hand, although best results are obtained with cameras having interchangeable waist-level viewfinders and ground glass screens. Use a cable release for all exposures. The adapter is attached to the camera in place of the lens. An eyepiece is removed from the camera and inserted into the adapter, which is then affixed over the microscope tube. The microscope image is viewed and focused through the camera's optical system.

Some experimentation will be needed to determine the appropriate color balance and exposure time. Tungsten-type films (balanced for indoor light) will work best with some light systems. If the light source has a rheostat, determine the optimum setting and use it consistently (color balance shifts toward blue with higher voltage). A voltage regulator may be used for consistent color balance. Use of a color filter may be necessary.

Exposure time may be determined by trial and error or by using the camera's built-in metering system. Bracketed exposures (calculated exposures, plus additional exposures one or two stops above and below) are often advisable. Some cameras which have only automatic exposure systems can be "fooled" into the correct exposure by setting the film speed indicator at half or double the actual sensitivity. Since exposures tend to be long, especially under high magnification, the microscope and camera must be placed on a firm surface in an area free of machinery and other vibrations. Be meticulous about focusing and adjusting the condenser lens system. Always close the microscope's diaphragm enough to keep stray light out of the optical path for maximum image sharpness. Store photographic slides in darkness in an atmosphere of relatively constant temperature and moderately low humidity.

THE ECONOMICS OF OFFICE LABORATORY TESTING

In-office hematology and blood chemistry testing with automated equipment can improve the quality of patient care by making results available quickly, often before the patient leaves the site. This is also advantageous from the marketing standpoint, since patients often appreciate quick answers and are favorably disposed toward practices that provide them. However, such testing should be undertaken only if it can be done with accurate results and if it is viable financially. The quality issue was discussed earlier in this chapter. The following factors should be considered in estimating the financial prospects:

1. What personnel are available to do the tests, either presently trained or capable and willing to learn?

2. What tests are being done presently? How often? Would the quality of care provided be enhanced by enlarging your test repertoire? How much are you paying for tests done through other laboratories? What reimbursement can be anticipated from patients and third parties if they are done on site?

3. What costs can be anticipated: capital or lease costs over a three- to five-year period? Supplies? Quality control? Other maintenance and repairs? Personnel time to obtain the specimens, perform the tests, and do accessory tasks such as record keeping and calibration? In some instances a decision may be made to do in-office testing for marketing purposes even though it is not expected to pay for itself.

4. What specific manufacturers and vendors should be invited to bring in equipment for trial? Information is often available from colleagues, local hospital personnel, advertisements, or through personal contacts with vendors at medical meetings.

Allow about two hours for an initial demonstration of the equipment. Have your personnel try running it. Ask about financing terms, guarantees, frequency and cost of calibration and quality control procedures, additional equipment or supplies needed, refrigerator or closet space needed for their storage, and shelf life of reagents both in unopened packages and after the seal has been broken. What resources are available for learning to use the system and for getting answers to questions that may arise during its use? How quickly and on what terms will service be available if a malfunction occurs? Be sure you have space for all elements of the system. Ask for references from practices presently using it.

Once the equipment is installed and in use, check to be sure that appropriate reimbursement is being received. Review procedure codes to be sure you are using the right ones. Keep a log of costs and relevant income to track them on a continuing basis.

SUGGESTED READING

Belsey R, Baer D, Sewell D: Laboratory test analysis near the patient: Opportunities for improved clinical diagnosis and management. *J Amer Med Assoc* 255:775, 1986.

Berg AO, Heidrich FE, Fihn SD, et al: Establishing the cause of genitourinary symptoms of women in a family practice: Comparison of clinical examination and comprehensive microbiology. *J Amer Med Assoc* 251:620, 1984.

Cartwright PS, Victory DF, Wong SW, et al: Evaluation of the new generation of urinary pregnancy tests. *Am J Obstet Gynecol* 153:730, 1985.

Fischer PM, Addison LA, Curtis P, et al: *The Office Laboratory.* Norwalk, Conn., Appleton-Century-Crofts, 1983.

Galen RS: Predictive value and efficiency of laboratory testing. *Ped Clin N Amer* 27(4):861, 1980.

Gillette RD: Streptococcal throat infections in family practice. *J Fam Pract* 6:251, 1978.

Jenkins RD, Fenn JP, Matsen JM: Review of urine microscopy for bacteriuria. *J Amer Med Assoc* 255:3397, 1986.

Jones JE: Office parasitology. *Am Fam Phys* 22(2):86, 1980.

MacDonald MJ: Personal blood glucose testing in children. *Pri Care* 10(4):565, 1983.

Miller RE, Paradise JL, Friday GA, et al: The nasal smear for eosinophils: Its value in children with seasonal allergic rhinitis. *Am J Dis Child* 136:1009, 1982.

Rich EC, Crowson TW, Connelly DP: Effectiveness of differential leukocyte count in case finding in the ambulatory care setting. *J Amer Med Assoc* 249:633, 1983.

Wardlaw SC, Levine RA: Quantitative buffy coat analysis: A new laboratory tool functioning as a screening complete blood cell count. *J Amer Med Assoc* 249:617, 1983.

chapter 18

Prescription Writing

The busy practitioner writes many prescriptions every working day, each of which has potential for either substantial benefit or serious harm to patient and doctor alike. If the preparation prescribed accomplishes its purpose, the patient benefits and the physician is put in a good light. If a significant error is made either in writing the prescription or in interpreting it, there may be adverse effects for the patient which may be reflected in subsequent criticism of or legal action against the doctor. A prescription is an order to dispense a certain drug in a certain way. This has important professional and legal consequences for both the doctor and the pharmacist. If the message is incomplete or unclear, the latter may misunderstand what was intended and dispense the wrong product or specify an incorrect dose. If the practitioner makes an error (and we all do, sooner or later) which the druggist does not recognize and question, the end result may be equally bad. The implications are clear: Write clearly, fill in all the blanks, double-check all entries for accuracy, and encourage local pharmacists to call promptly if they have any questions about your instructions. Physicians with worse-than-average handwriting should consider printing or typing their prescriptions.

Prescription forms are usually custom-printed for each practice in the standard $4\frac{1}{4}$- by $5\frac{1}{2}$-inch size (figure 18-1). The name, address, and telephone number of the practice appear at the top. The names of all physicians in the practice (and other professionals, if authorized to write prescriptions) may be listed unless there are too many of them for the available space. There are spaces for the date and the patient's name, address, and age. The address must be included in prescriptions for controlled substances and is always desirable because it would help the pharmacist locate the patient in case of a drug recall or other unanticipated problem with the prescription. In many larger practices this information can all be put on a plastic address stamp plate and stamped in an area provided for this purpose on the top-right corner of the form.

The space for the name and quantity of the drug being prescribed is in the middle of the form. The drug name and dosage form are written on one line, and the amount to be dispensed on the next. Use standard metric units of measurement. Check when in doubt to be sure that a drug you wish to prescribe is available in the dosage form you have in mind.

Instructions to the patient are written just below this, preferably behind

---

AVONDALE FAMILY PHYSICIANS

7700 First Avenue
Cincinnati, Ohio 54321
Tel. 123–4567

06-17-86
WILSON, MARY J.
3719 FOREST STREET
CINCINNATI OH 54321
H/H EDGAR BC/BS
DOB 3/7/49

R

Aspirin with codeine 30 mgm tablets
#20 (twenty)

Sig: Take one or two tablets q 4h for pain

Refill ____ X 1 ____

Label Contents

M. B. Jones MD

DEA# AJ 1234567

DRS. REDD, WHITE & BLEU, P.C.
FAMILY PHYSICIANS

1234 Fifth Avenue   Tel. 987–6543

Name Mary Smith   Age 12

Address 2345 Rose Lane

R   Amoxicillin Suspension 250 mg/5 ml.
150 ml.

SIG: 1 teaspoon before breakfast, after
school, and at bedtime until gone

R.U. Bleu MD

Refill n.r.   DEA#____

FIGURE 18-1
Sample prescriptions.

the letters "Sig:" an indication that what follows is the "signa," or directions for taking the medicine. To maximize compliance, try to tie pill-taking times to customary daily activities such as meals or coming home from work or school. If there is risk that a patient may discontinue a drug such as an antibiotic before the prescribed course of treatment is finished, specify that it is to be taken "until gone." Avoid indefinite phrases such as "take as directed." If the instructions are too long to fit on the prescription label, write them out for the patient and have the bottle labeled "take according to written instructions." Druggists often dispense excellent printed directions supplied by pharmaceutical manufacturers. It's helpful to keep these and other educational materials on hand in the office for patients who need information either about the effects of drugs or the method of using them. With most patients a combination of verbal and printed instructions is more effective than either alone.

Many misunderstandings have arisen from the inappropriate use of abbreviations in prescription writing. Some authors believe that all instructions should be written out in English, but the following traditional abbreviations of Latin phrases are acceptable:

ac (*ante cibum*)	before meals
bid (*bis in die*)	twice daily
hs (*hora somni*)	at bedtime
nr (*non repitatur*)	do not repeat
pc (*post cibum*)	after meals
prn (*pro re nata*)	as needed
qid (*quarter in die*)	four times daily
q__h (*quaque__hora*)	every__hours
tid (*ter in die*)	three times daily

The common abbreviations "qd" and "qod," signifying "every day" and "every other day," respectively, are best avoided because they can easily be confused with "qid."

There is a line at the bottom right for the practitioner's signature; the letters "M.D." may be printed at the end. A line for entry of the doctor's Drug Enforcement Agency (DEA) registration number should be included since it is required for controlled substance prescriptions. Pharmacists put the name and strength of the drug on the container label routinely, but the phrase "Label contents" may be printed in the lower-left corner as confirmation that this should be done. It can be crossed out in the occasional circumstance where the doctor wants that information omitted.

Special thought should be given to the subject of refill instructions because they have a significant impact on one's practice and relationship with patients. Writing appropriate refill instructions on the prescription can save time, telephone calls, and aggravation for the busy physician. If a short-term illness is being treated or there is significant concern about safety, the pharmacist may be instructed not to refill the order (the abbreviation "nr" will convey this message). If the circumstances are such that self-treatment carries little risk, the practitioner may decide to authorize one or two refills.

When treating a reliable patient for a chronic illness, one may choose to make the prescription refillable until a certain date, such as January 1 of the next year. Prescriptions other than for controlled substances may be made refillable indefinitely, although this sometimes leads to perennial use of drugs by patients without adequate physician supervision. A good way to accomplish these goals is to put a line, "Refill ____" at the lower-left corner of the blank, for entries such as "nr," "x2," "until 1 Jan. ____" or whatever else may be appropriate.

Keeping accurate prescription records is important for both medical and legal reasons. Trying to remember how many of what kind of pills have been prescribed for which patients is unrealistic for most physicians and totally unworkable in a facility where numerous practitioners may be involved in the care of individual patients. The use of duplicate prescription forms is desirable from a legal standpoint but is cumbersome in settings where many prescriptions are generated. The most practical approach is to note precisely what was ordered for each patient in the clinical note. A typical entry might read, "Prescribed penicillin V K tablets 250 mg, #30, to be taken 1 tid until they are gone, nr."

There are a number of steps one can take to minimize the risk of prescription drug abuse. Keep prescription pads under lock and key, not on a desktop or in a drawer accessible by patients who are alone in an examining room. Use colored and perhaps patterned paper that is difficult to photocopy. Fill in DEA registration numbers only when they are needed, rather than printing them on the prescription form. Do not sign blank forms to be completed later by a nurse. Write in ink rather than pencil. To keep a patient from adding a zero to the end of the number of pills you have instructed the pharmacist to dispense, draw a circle tightly around the number or, better yet, write the number out, as for example "tablets #30 (thirty)." Avoid habituating drugs when others can be substituted safely. Be suspicious about unfamiliar patients with stories that seem to require you to prescribe controlled drugs. Let it be known to local pharmacists that you want them to call whenever they feel uncomfortable about filling a prescription you have written; they may know of patients who are getting controlled drugs from more than one doctor or have other information you can use to help avoid abuse of prescribed drugs.

In a busy practice there is often a temptation to telephone prescription orders to druggists or to delegate this responsibility to members of the office staff. Before doing so one needs to be familiar with relevant state and federal regulations and have clear guidelines as to what staff members with various levels of training and experience will be permitted to do. Accurate record keeping by everyone involved is essential. It is important not to let patients keep refilling prescriptions without periodic recheck visits to the physician.

One additional benefit of accurate clinical records is their ability to guide the doctor in assessing patient compliance. If, for example, a patient who was given a prescription for twenty capsules with instructions to take one capsule three times daily still has half of them left at the next visit seven days later, simple arithmetic indicates that the medicine has not been taken regularly. Be cautious about confronting the patient with this information, though, because that could create ill-will and make it difficult to obtain similar information in the future.

SUGGESTED READING

Ingrim NB, Hokanson JA, Guernsey BG, et al: Physician noncompliance with prescription-writing requirements. *Am J Hosp Pharm* 40:414, 1983.

U.S. Department of Justice, Drug Enforcement Administration: *Physician's Manual: An Informational Outline of the Controlled Substances Act of 1970.* Washington, D.C., Drug Enforcement Administration, revised 1985.

chapter 19

Equipment and Supplies

Office-based primary care utilizes a large variety of equipment and supplies, with significant variation from one practice to another based on patient volume, types of procedures done, personal interests and preferences of the physician(s), physical arrangement of the building, and other variables. The following list assumes a very busy one-doctor primary care practice or a two- to five-doctor practice in a setting where subspecialists are not readily available "down the hall." Height and weight measurements are assumed to be done before the patients enter the examining rooms; blood pressures and temperatures are checked in the rooms. Minor surgery and other more significant procedures are performed in a treatment room established for that purpose. Audiometry and vision testing are done in a multipurpose diagnostic room; electrocardiography and spirometry can be done there as well, or for convenience the equipment can be rolled to examining rooms on carts. Seldom-used equipment and supplies are stored in or near a central nurses station. Blood for laboratory testing can be drawn either in the examining rooms or at the office laboratory.

The list which follows should be considered a point of departure which readers can use as a guide to their own choices. Many physicians starting practice may elect to acquire only selected items at first, adding others as their practices grow. Some may prefer alternate purchases which may prove equally satisfactory.

EXAMINING ROOM EQUIPMENT

Examining table with adjustable upper section, disappearing leg rest, and multiple storage drawers (Heated drawer for vaginal specula is desirable.)

Floor-mounted examining light with focused quartz light source and gooseneck adjustment (A wall- or ceiling-mounted light is desirable but more expensive. A head-mounted ENT examining light is a useful, relatively inexpensive option for vaginal and other endoscopic examinations.)

Two side chairs

Roll-around stool, adjustable height

Waste disposal unit; may be built-in

Storage cabinets; often built-in

Small writing desk; may be built-in or wall-mounted

Hand-held mirror for patient's use during pelvic examinations

128-Hz tuning fork for vibratory testing

1056-Hz tuning fork for hearing screening

Reflex hammer

Large safety pin or Wartenburg pinwheel for testing skin sensation

Otoscope-ophthalmoscope set with pneumatic otoscope bulb and tubing; may be wall-mounted

Sphygmomanometer with detachable cuffs of various sizes; may be wall-mounted

Vaginal specula, sizes virginal, small, medium, and large; Graves and/or Pederson patterns (Metal specula preferred by most physicians, although some use disposable plastic ones.)

Fetoscope (or Doppler fetoscope shared among rooms and kept at nurses station)

EXAMINING ROOM SUPPLIES

Examining gowns or capes; may be disposable

Sheets; may be disposable

Disposable unsterile examining gloves

Water-soluble surgical lubricant (K-Y, etc.)

Box of facial tissue

Endocervical aspiration sets, disposable

Microscope slides, 1 × 3 inches, frosted end

Microscope coverslips

30% potassium hydroxide solution in dropper bottle

Normal saline solution in dropper bottle

Sterile applicators, one or two in an envelope

Calcium alginate sterile swabs

$\frac{3}{4}$- × 3-inch and 1- × 3-inch adhesive strip bandages

Disposable ruled measuring tapes

Disposable plastic anoscopes

Disposable medicine cups, 15 or 30 ml

Tongue depressors, unwrapped

Cervical scrapers, wood, extended tip

Pap test preservative spray or hair spray (see chapter 12)

Candida culture medium, Microstix Candida or Nickerson's medium

Disposable otoscope specula, adult and pediatric sizes

Test kits and developer for fecal occult blood tests

Disposable alcohol swabs

Unsterile 2- × 2-inch gauze squares

Disposable urine specimen containers (stored here or elsewhere, as preferred)

Podophylline 20% in compound tincture of benzoin

Ethyl chloride or other freezing spray

Flexible collodion

Menstrual pads and tampons

If Dressing Changes Are Done Here

Suture removal sets, disposable or reusable

Sterile scissors

Sterile dressing forceps

Bandage scissors

Sterile gauze squares, 3- × 3- and 4- × 4-inch sizes

Paper adhesive tape, 0.5-, 1-, and 2-inch widths

Flexible roller gauze, 1- and 2-inch widths

Sterile examining/surgical gloves

Compound tincture of benzoin or proprietary skin adhesive such as Mastisol (liquid and/or pressurized spray)

Elastic bandages, 2- and 3-inch sizes; self-adherent type such as Coban suggested

Nonstick inner dressing pads (Telfa, Adaptic, or other), small sizes, sterile

Wound closure strips, sterile, $\frac{1}{8}$- and $\frac{1}{4}$-inch widths (Steri-strips, others)

Silver nitrate sticks

If Diagnostic Blood Drawing Is Done Here

Tourniquets

Finger lancets, disposable; use of spring lancet optional

Microhematocrit tubes

Microhematocrit tube sealant putty

Vacuum blood drawing equipment:
- regular and sleeved needles
- various sizes and types of blood tubes
- plastic holder for needles and tubes

Hand-held glucose meter (may be stored at nurses station)

Glucose test strips

NURSES STATION

Storage cabinets, sink, and desk space; usually built-in

Locked cabinet for controlled drugs

Refrigerator (undercounter type usually sufficient)

Adult scales with device for measuring height

Pediatric scales or pediatric table with built-in scale and system for measuring length

Emesis basins

Prep basins, small and large

Large foot and forearm basins

Equipment for disposing of used syringes, needles, and surgical blades

Ear syringe or pulsed dental water-jet pump with ear-irrigating tip

Ear irrigation basin, Goldnamer pattern

Large plastic aprons for ear syringing and treatment of nosebleed

Doppler instrument for fetal and/or peripheral vessel examinations (optional)

Set of vaginal test diaphragms or fitting rings

Disposable hypodermic syringes, 3 ml, with 25-gauge $\times \frac{5}{8}$-inch and 22-gauge $\times 1\frac{1}{4}$-inch needles

Disposable tuberculin syringes with 26-gauge $\times \frac{3}{8}$-inch and 25-gauge $\times \frac{5}{8}$-inch needles

Disposable 6-ml and 12-ml hypodermic syringes

Disposable hypodermic needles, 18-gauge $\times 1\frac{1}{2}$-inch, 20-gauge $\times 1\frac{1}{2}$-inch, 22-gauge $\times 1\frac{1}{2}$-inch, 27-gauge $\times$ 1-inch sizes

Disposable alcohol swabs

Injectable drugs including immunizing agents, analgesics, sedatives, antibiotics, corticosteroids, anticholinergics, epinephrine, others at physician's option

Drops for softening earwax (see chapter 7 regarding Cerumenex drops)

Cotton balls, unsterile

Instrument for relieving subungual hematomas; battery-powered small cautery device recommended

Ring cutter

5-foot piece of sturdy string for removing rings from swollen fingers

Toenail nippers

"Air splints" for ankles and forearms

Infant, child, adult, and oversize blood pressure cuffs to use with sphygmomanometers in the examining rooms.

2-inch cloth adhesive tape for strapping ankle sprains

Dome-paste or Gelocast dressing material for Unna Boot dressings

Toluene (for pinworm diagnosis)

Mineral oil (for scabies diagnosis, other uses)

Monsel's or aluminum chloride solution for topical hemostasis

Solution for removing adhesive tape residues (acetone is effective, although flammable)

Paper drinking cups

Examining table paper rolls

In Refrigerator

Various biologicals (some will need to be stored frozen)

Culture media for throat, gonococcal, and other cultures

Drugs which require refrigeration

Eye Tray

Binocular loupe or other magnifier as preferred

Source of violet light

Schiotz tonometer

Eye magnet (optional)

Toothpicks with small amounts of cotton batting on ends, sterilized, for ocular foreign bodies

Applicator sticks to assist in everting eyelids

Eye-irrigating solution, large squeeze bottle

(Topical anesthetic such as 0.5% tetracaine, stored in refrigerator unless single-use units are employed)

Sterile eye pads

1-inch paper or clear-plastic adhesive tape

Metal eye shields

Mydriatic solution such as tropicamide or 2.5% phenylephrine

Other topical drugs as preferred by physicians

ENT Tray

Large bayonet thumb forceps

Small angulated thumb forceps, Wilde pattern

Articulated foreign body forceps, Noyes or similar

Bivalve nasal speculae, Vienna pattern, large and small

#3 and #5 laryngeal mirrors

Self-illuminated laryngeal telescope (optional)

Set of oval ear specula, Brown or Gruber pattern

Malleable metal ear applicator

Ear spoons or curettes

Alcohol lamp or solution for defogging laryngeal mirrors

Cotton balls or pledgets

Head mirror or focused head-mounted examining light

Small suction cannula with thumb-operated relief valve, Baron pattern or similar

Unsterile 4- × 4-inch gauze squares

(Epinephrine 1:1000, ampules or small bottle, kept in refrigerator)

DIAGNOSTIC ROOM

Electrocardiograph machine on roll-around stand

Supply of ruled paper to fit ECG machine

Electrode paste

Electrode pads (optional)

Examining gowns or capes

Spirometer on roll-around stand

Supply of ruled paper to fit spirometer

Disposable mouthpieces

Note: It will often be convenient to take the ECG machine to a patient who is already disrobed in an examining room; at other times, especially if the examining rooms are busy, one may elect to do the procedure in the diagnostic room. The same considerations may apply to spirometry.

Peak-flow spirometer, hand-held (The Mini-Wright or similar instrument is often useful in following the course of reactive airways disease.)

Audiometer (ideally, in a soundproof booth)

Impedance tympanometer (optional)

Ultrasound or diathermy treatment unit (optional)

A special contact gel, used with ultrasound treatment

Vision testing machine (Keystone, Titmus, other)

Alternate approach: wall-mounted Snellen eye chart, illiterate E wall chart, hand-held cardboard near-vision testing chart, and Ishihara pseudoisochromatic plate book for color testing

TREATMENT/SURGERY ROOM

Table with height, Trendelenburg, and proctoscopic adjustments

Arm boards

Papoose board

Ceiling-mounted examining/operating light

Cart with defibrillator and drugs and supplies for cardiopulmonary resuscitation

Portable emergency oxygen equipment

Mayo stand

Flexible sigmoidoscope with accessories

Suction pump (Electric is preferred; water-powered aspirator acceptable; in either case be sure there is an adequate suction bottle in the system to keep aspirated materials out of the pump.)

Suction tubing, disposable

Suction catheters and tips

Waste containers with plastic liners

Adjustable roll-around stool

Step stool for use by patients

Floor stand or ceiling hook for intravenous infusions

Small electrosurgery unit (Hyfrecator, other brands)

Cryotherapy unit, nitrous oxide-powered (optional)

Bandage scissors

Transfer forceps set

Instrument tray with lid

Contents of Instrument Tray

Iris scissors or small suture-removal scissors

Larger dissecting scissors

Malleable blunt probe

Extra thumb forceps, dressing pattern

Comedo extractor

Skin biopsy punches, if not using disposable type

Note: Keeping instruments in a covered tray soaking in a germicidal solution gives less reliable sterility than autoclaving, but the latter may be unsatisfactory for sharp-edged instruments susceptible to rusting. Scissors may be autoclaved if absolute sterility is judged more important than possible loss of sharpness.

Suture Sets

Needle holder, 5-inch, smooth beveled jaws
Tissue forceps, Adson or similar
3 mosquito hemostats, curved or straight as preferred
#3 scalpel handle, if using disposable blades only
gauze squares, 3- × 3-inch size

Supplemental Surgical Set

Small self-retaining retractors
2 Allis clamps
3 larger hemostats
3 spring-type towel clips
2 skin hooks
3 sterile towels

Gynecology Set

Single-tooth tenaculum
Uterine dressing forceps
Malleable uterine sound
Cervical biopsy punch
Fluffed gauze pads

Individually Wrapped Sterile Instruments

Set of 3 mosquito hemostats
Needle holder
Dressing forceps
Tissue forceps
Needle holder–scissors combination (optional; for rapid repair of minor lacerations)
Splinter forceps, Virtus or similar

4- and 6-mm skin biopsy punches (may be disposable type)

Bone rongeur

Large curved forceps for pharyngeal foreign bodies

Small prep basin with 3- × 3-inch gauze squares

Intravenous Infusion Supplies

1000-ml containers of normal saline, 5% glucose, and balanced electrolyte solutions; others as desired

Infusion tubing sets

Intravenous catheters, 18 and 20 gauge

Scalp vein infusion sets

Other Sterile Supplies

Disposable fenestrated drapes for suturing and minor surgical procedures

Antistick dressing materials (Adaptic, Telfa, etc., in various sizes)

Suture materials on 3/8 circle-cutting needles: 4/0 and 5/0 monofilament nylon or polypropylene, and 4/0 polyglycolate; other sizes as preferred by physicians

Disposable scalpels or scalpel blades, #15 and #12 patterns, others as desired

Gauze pads, 3- × 3- and 4- × 4-inch sizes

Rolled dressings, 1-, 2-, 3-inch and wider sizes (Kling, Kerlix, other brands)

Sterile wound closure strips, $\frac{1}{8}$- and $\frac{1}{4}$-inch widths (Steri-strips, etc.)

Sterile surgical gloves, prepackaged in pairs

3-ml disposable hypodermic syringes with 25-gauge × $\frac{5}{8}$-inch and 22-gauge × $1\frac{1}{4}$-inch needles

6- and 12-ml hypodermic syringes

20-gauge × $1\frac{1}{2}$-inch hypodermic needles

18-gauge × $1\frac{1}{2}$-inch hypodermic needles

27-gauge × 1-inch hypodermic needles

Soft rubber drain material, Penrose drain or pieces cut to shape from surgical gloves

Orthopedic Equipment and Supplies

Electric cast cutter

Cast spreader

Indelible pencil for marking casts

2-, 3-, and 4-inch plaster rolls, extra-fast setting

Packaged plaster splint material (optional)

3-inch sheet wadding

Stockinette rolls, 3-inch (optional)

Slings, assorted sizes

Rib belts, assorted sizes

Elastic bandages, 2-, 3-, and 4-inch width (self-adherent type such as Coban suggested)

Foam-backed aluminum finger splint material, to be cut to size with bandage scissors (Alumafoam, etc.)

"Frog" splints for sprained fingers

Other assorted aluminum finger splints

Adjustable crutches, child and adult sizes

Miscellaneous

Spray dressing material (Aeroplast, etc.)

Liquid and/or spray skin adherent (Mastisol, compound tincture of benzoin)

Disposable cold packs

10% formalin in small bottles, with labels, for tissue specimen preservation

Iodophor or chlorhexidine scrub solution

Lidocaine 0.5% with epinephrine

Lidocaine 1.0% without epinephrine

Bupivacaine 0.25%

Note: The added expense of knee- or foot-operated faucets is amply repaid over the useful life of the fixtures. The sink should be large enough for comfortable surgical scrubbing. If much cast work is done, its drain should be equipped with a plaster trap.

Laboratory Equipment

Microscope with dustcover

Incubator, countertop

Refrigerator, undercounter

Fire extinguisher, wall-mounted (Mount it a few feet away from places where a fire could start.)

Alcohol or Bunsen burner

Microhematocrit centrifuge

Angle-head clinical centrifuge

Rack and tubes for Westergren sedimentation rate test

Proprietary instruments for automated blood cell counts and chemistry determinations (optional)

Alternatives: Hemocytometer with coverslip, prepackaged diluting units for WBC counts (Unopette, etc.), Spencer hemoglobinometer with hemolysis sticks

Urinometer with extra floats

Alternative: Refractometer

Slide-staining tray

Slide-holding forceps

Bacteriologist's loop

Log books

Laboratory Supplies

Sterile sheep blood agar plates

Bacitracin identification disks for group A streptococci

Culture or transfer media for GC cultures

Urine collection containers

Other sterile specimen containers

Disposable centrifuge tubes

Long disposable pipettes with bulbs

Lens paper

Xylene or proprietary lens cleaning solution

Multiple-test urine dipsticks

Urine sediment-staining solution (Sedistain, etc.; optional)

Wright's or Giemsa's stain set

Gram stain set

Plastic wash bottle for staining procedures

Supplies for blood drawing (see "Examining Room Equipment" section above)

Commercial Laboratory Test Kits

Serum pregnancy test

Urine pregnancy test

Urine culturing

Infectious mononucleosis

Rapid group A streptoccal identification

Equipment and Supplies for Sterilization

Counter-mounted autoclave with time and pressure indicators

Sterile wraps of various sizes

Sterilization envelopes of various sizes

Autoclave tape with indicator stripes

Tube-type sterilization indicators

Distilled water, gallons

Detergent and brushes for cleaning equipment

Instrument germicide solution with rust inhibitor (Cidex, etc.)

Note: The technique of cleaning and sterilizing equipment is important. See first reference under "Suggested Reading."

SUGGESTED READING

Cooper MG, Cooper DE: *The Medical Assistant,* 5th ed. New York, McGraw-Hill, 1986, pp. 315–339.

Nazarian LF: The well-equipped office, in Green M, Haggerty RJ (ed): *Ambulatory Pediatrics III.* Philadelphia, Saunders, 1984, pp. 509–520.

Robinson DW: Planning a private office, in Taylor RB (ed): *Family Medicine: Principles and Practice,* 2d ed. New York, Springer-Verlag, 1983, pp. 1749–1765.

Index